Blueprints

Clinical Cases in Pediatrics

Blueprints
Clinical Cases
in Pediatrics

Vedang A. Londhe, MD

Andrea K. Marmor, MD

Abhay S. Dandekar, MD

Aaron B. Caughey, MD, MPP, MPH (Series Editor)

Blackwell
Publishing

© 2002 by Blackwell Science, Inc.
a Blackwell Publishing Company

Editorial Offices:
Commerce Place, 350 Main Street, Malden, Massachusetts 02148, USA
Osney Mead, Oxford OX2 0EL, England
25 John Street, London WC1N 2BS, England
23 Ainslie Place, Edinburgh EH3 6AJ, Scotland
54 University Street, Carlton, Victoria 3053, Australia

Other Editorial Offices:
Blackwell Wissenschafts-Verlag GmbH, Kurfürstendamm 57, 10707 Berlin, Germany
Blackwell Science KK, MG Kodenmacho Building, 7-10 Kodenmacho
   Nihombashi, Chuo-ku, Tokyo 104, Japan
Iowa State University Press, A Blackwell Science Company, 2121 S. State Avenue,
   Ames, Iowa 50014-8300, USA

Distributors:

The Americas
   Blackwell Publishing
   c/o AIDC
   P.O. Box 20
   50 Winter Sport Lane
   Williston, VT 05495-0020
   (Telephone orders: 800-216-2522;
   fax orders: 802-864-7626)

Australia
   Blackwell Science Pty, Ltd.
   54 University Street
   Carlton, Victoria 3053
   (Telephone orders: 03-9347-0300;
   fax orders: 03-9349-3016)

Outside The Americas and Australia
   Blackwell Science, Ltd.
   c/o Marston Book Services, Ltd.
   P.O. Box 269
   Abingdon
   Oxon OX14 4YN
   England
   (Telephone orders: 44-01235-465500;
   fax orders: 44-01235-465555)

Acquisitions: Beverly Copland
Development: Angela Gagliano
Production: Jennifer Kowalewski
Manufacturing: Lisa Flanagan
Marketing Manager: Kathleen Mulcahy
Cover design: Hannus Design
Interior design: Julie Gallagher
Typeset by International Typesetting and Composition
Printed and bound by Capital City Press

Printed in the United States of America
02 03 04 05 5 4 3 2 1

Library of Congress Cataloging-in-Publication Data

Blueprints clinical cases in pediatrics / by Vedang A. Londhe ...[et al.].
      p. ; cm. — (Blueprints clinical cases)
   ISBN 0-632-04605-8 (pbk.)
   1. Pediatrics—Case studies.
   [DNLM: 1. Pediatrics—Case Report. 2. Pediatrics—Examination Questions.
WS 18.2 B6578 2002] I. Londhe, Vedang A. II. Series.
   RJ58 .B58 2002
   618.92'00076–dc21   2002000692

Notice: The indications and dosages of all drugs in this book have been recommended in the medical literature and conform to the practices of the general community. The medications described and treatment prescriptions suggested do not necessarily have specific approval by the Food and Drug Administration for use in the diseases and dosages for which they are recommended. The package insert for each drug should be consulted for use and dosage as approved by the FDA. Because standards for usage change, it is advisable to keep abreast of revised recommendations, particularly those concerning new drugs.

AUTHORS

Vedang A. Londhe, MD
   University of California, Los Angeles
   Los Angeles, California

Andrea K. Marmor, MD
   Fellow in General Pediatrics
   University of California, San Francisco
   San Francisco, California

Abhay S. Dandekar, MD
   Chief Resident, Department of Pediatrics
   Kaiser Permanente Medical Center
   Oakland, California

Aaron B. Caughey, MD, MPP, MPH (Series Editor)
   Fellow in Maternal-Fetal Medicine
   Department of Obstetrics and Gynecology
   University of California, San Francisco
   San Francisco, California

DEDICATION

For my son, Shaan, and his mom, Anjali
Ved

I would like to dedicate my portion of this book to the many people who have inspired me to learn and to teach every day of my life. From the patients, students and physicians who constantly challenge me to become a better doctor, to my friends and family who are my teachers in life, I extend to each of you credit for this book, my warmest thanks, and the joy of lifelong learning.
Andi

I would like to thank my wife, Aparna, for her unwavering support. I would also like to thank my teachers and colleagues for continuously nurturing my desire to learn.
Abhay

We would all like to thank the staff at Blackwell Publishing particularly Bev Copland and Angela Gagliano for their untiring work on this project. We would also like to thank our family, friends and colleagues including the residents and faculty in the Departments of Pediatrics and Obstetrics and Gynecology at UCSF, Kaiser Oakland, and UCLA. I dedicate this book to my parents, Bill and Carol, who have had an immeasurable effect on the children they have cared for throughout their careers.
Aaron

CONTENTS

CONTENTS

PREFACE

Blueprints Clinical Cases in Pediatrics was developed to enrich and supplement the clinical experience of the medical student or sub-intern rotating through pediatrics. We have designed and written these problem-based scenarios to emphasize the most common and important childhood illnesses, as well as to hit hot topics that will appear on in-service examinations, on rounds, and on Boards.

The cases also reflect the special challenges of the diagnosis and treatment of illness in children. As you know, children are not simply small adults, and many of the diseases and conditions that affect infants and children are unique. In addition, the unusual and often subtle presentation of disease in pediatric patients demands patience and attention to details such as vital signs, growth parameters, and the interaction between the parent and child.

Case-based learning is fun and effective, but requires substantial motivation from the student for maximum benefit. The cases are designed to take you through the clinical thought process, beginning with the patient's complaint, proceeding through history, exam and diagnostic tests, and ending with diagnosis and management. As you work through the cases, focus on improving your skills in assessment of the sick child, as well as making the diagnosis and learning about the specific illness. The following are suggestions on how to get the most out of the pediatric cases.

1. **Approach the cases as you approach your patients.** Read the information carefully, pay attention to details, and think about what you would ask or do next.
2. **Write down your answers to the Thought Questions before moving on.** This is a key step in maximizing your learning from the cases. In the interest of space we have presented only pertinent positives and negatives. If a portion of the history or physical exam that you are interested in is not presented, assume it to be normal or noncontributory (but it should still be a part of your complete history and physical!).
3. **Note the elements of the history that are unique to pediatrics.** These include the birth history, immunization history and developmental history. This information is presented when relevant to the case, and should be carefully reviewed. Social and family histories are also important in pediatrics, as children depend on their caretakers for adequate nutrition, injury prevention, and other health maintenance behaviors.
4. **Pay special attention to the vital signs and growth parameters in each case.** Since children often cannot communicate to us about discomfort or distress, abnormal vital signs are an important clue to the etiology of illness, and may be the only abnormalities on physical exam. The vital signs presented are normal for age unless a range of values appears after them, and percentiles are given for all growth parameters.
5. **Assess the nutritional status and hydration of the child.** Plot each child's height and weight on the growth curve in the back of the book. Look for evidence of hydration status on history and physical exam, such as fluid intake, urine output, tachycardia, mucous membranes, skin color and capillary refill.
6. **Answer the multiple choice questions at the end of each case.** These questions and answers provide additional important information about the case diagnosis, and address additional conditions in the differential that are worth knowing about.
7. **Read about topics that you want to know more about in** Blueprints **in Pediatrics, or in a pediatric textbook.** You can also do a literature search to find out about recent discoveries and current therapy for topics that interest you.
8. **Remember that pediatrics, like all of medicine, is a constantly changing field.** Check with the pediatricians that you are working with to find out the latest information on diagnosis and treatment.

We hope that you find the pediatric cases fun and interesting, and a good complement to your experience in the pediatric clinic, nursery and ward. Keep your eyes and ears open, children have a lot to teach us all!

Vedang A. Londhe, MD
Andrea K. Marmor, MD
Abhay S. Dandekar, MD

ABBREVIATIONS/ACRONYMS

ABC	airway, breathing, circulation
ABD	abdomen
ABG	arterial blood gas
AFOSF	anterior fontanel open/soft/flat
AIDS	acquired immunodeficiency syndrome
All	Allergies
ALL	acute lymphocytic leukemia
AN	anorexia nervosa
ANA	antinuclear antibody
ARF	acute rheumatic fever
ASD	atrial septal defect
BP	blood pressure
BUN	blood urea nitrogen
C	Celsius
CAH	congenital adrenal hyperplasia
CCAM	congenital cystadenomatous malformations
C/C/E	cyanosis/clubbing/edema
CBC	complete blood count
CC/ID	chief complaint/identification
CDC	Centers for Disease Control
CM	costal margin
CMV	cytomegalovirus
CNS	central nervous system
CPAP	continuous positive airway pressure
CRP	C-reactive protein
CRT	capillary refill time
CSF	cerebrospinal fluid
CT	computerized tomography
CTA(B)	clear to auscultation (bilaterally)
CV	cardiovascular
CXR	chest x-ray
DKA	diabetic ketoacidosis
DMSA	dimercaptosuccinic acid
DOL	day of life
DTR	deep tendon reflex
EBV	Epstein-Barr virus
ECG/EKG	electrocardiogram
ED/ER	emergency department (room)
EEG	electroencephalogram
EOMI	extraocular movements intact
ESR	erythrocyte sedimentation rate
F	Fahrenheit
FRC	functional residual capacity
FTT	failure to thrive
GAS	Group A *Streptococcus*
GBM	glomerular basement membrane
GBS	Guillain-Barré syndrome
GERD	gastroesophageal reflux disease
GI	gastrointestinal
GN	glomerulonephritis
GU	genitourinary
HEENT	head, eyes, ears, nose, throat
HHV	human herpesvirus
HIV	human immunodeficiency virus
HLA	human leukocyte antigen
HPI	history of present illness

HSP	Henoch-Schönlein purpura
HSV	herpes simplex virus
IBD	inflammatory bowel disease
ICH	intracranial hemorrhage
ICN	intensive care nursery
ICP	intracranial pressure
IDDM	insulin-dependent diabetes mellitus
ITP	idiopathic thrombocytopenic purpura
IV	intravenous
IVIG	intravenous immunoglogulin
IVP	intravenous pyelogram
JRA	juvenile rheumatoid arthritis
KUB	kidney ureters bladder (radiograph)
LLQ	left lower quadrant
LP	lumbar puncture
LR	Lactated Ringer's solution
LUQ	left upper quadrant
LVH	left ventricular hypertrophy
MAP	mean arterial pressure
MCD	minimal change disease
MRI	magnetic resonance imaging
MS	musculoskeletal
NABS	normal active bowel sounds
NAD	no acute distress
NCAT	normocephalic atraumatic
ND	non-distended
NHL	non-Hodgkin lymphomas
NICU	neonatal intensive care unit
NKDA	no known drug allergy
NS	normal saline
NSAID	nonsteroidal anti-inflammatory drugs
NSVD	normal spontaneous vaginal delivery
NT	non-tender
OP	oropharynx
OR	operating room
OTC	over-the-counter
P	pulse
PE	physical exam
PERRLA	pupils equal round/reactive to light/accommodation
PICU	pediatric intensive care unit
PID	pelvic inflammatory disease
PMHx	past medical history
PPD	purified protein derivative
PPHN	persistent pulmonary hypertension
PRN	as needed
PSGN	poststreptococcal glomerulonephritis
PSurgHx	past surgical history
PT/PTT	prothrombin time/partial thromboplastin time
RA	room air
RAD	reactive airway disease
RBC	red blood cell
RDS	respiratory distress syndrome
Resp	respiratory/respirations
RLQ	right lower quadrant
ROS	review of systems

RR	respiratory rate		TORCH	Toxoplasma, Other (syphilis, HIV, EBV), Rubella, CMV, Herpes
RR&R	regular rate and rhythm		UA	urinalysis
RSV	respiratory syncytial virus		UC	ulcerative colitis
RUQ	right upper quadrant		U/S	ultrasound
RVH	right ventricular quadrant		URI	upper respiratory infection
SCFE	slipped capital femoral epiphysis		UTD	up to date
SHx	social history		UTI	urinary tract infection
SLE	systemic lupus erythematosus		VCUG	voiding cystourethrogram
STD	sexually transmitted disease		VDRL	venereal disease reference laboratory
SVD	spontaneous vaginal delivery		VS	vitals signs
SVT	supraventricular tachycardia		VSD	ventricular septal defect
T	temperature		WBC	white blood cell
TAPVR	total anomalous pulmonary venous return		WNL	within normal limits
TGA	transposition of the great arteries		WPW	Woff-Parkinson-White
TM	tympanic membrane		Wt	weight

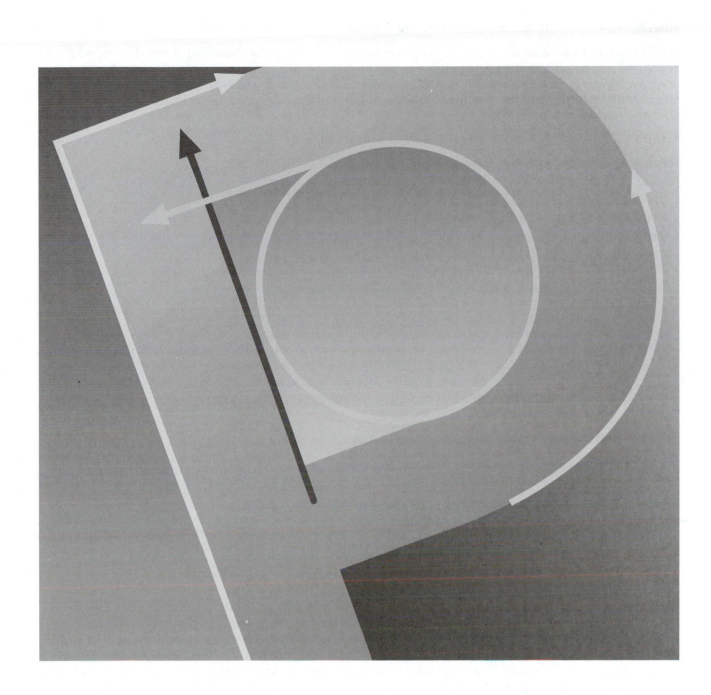

CASES

CASE 1 / FEVER AND FUSSINESS

ID/CC: 16-month-old girl brought in by her mother for fussiness and fever.

HPI: O.M. has had a cold for 3 days, with runny nose and cough, and last night she developed a fever and increased fussiness. She refuses to eat and only wants her bottle. Last night O.M. woke up crying and was inconsolable until she got ibuprofen for fever, and was finally able to go back to sleep. Mother says she acted like this 3 months ago when she had an ear infection, and she is worried that she has one again.

PMHx: Ear infection 4 months ago; resolved with treatment.

Meds: Ibuprofen for fever   **All:** None   **Immunizations:** Up to date (UTD)

THOUGHT QUESTIONS

- What illnesses besides ear infection are you considering at this point?
- What findings will you look for in this child's ear to confirm the diagnosis of ear infection?

Although this child most likely has an upper respiratory infection, you should always consider more serious infections like pneumonia and meningitis in the febrile and irritable child. Always evaluate the child's hydration status and carefully examine the lungs, skin, joints, and nervous system for signs of focal bacterial infection. As always in the child aged 3 to 36 months, consider a workup for occult bacteremia or urinary tract infection (UTI) if a source for the fever cannot be found. In an older child who complains of ear pain, otitis externa ("swimmer's ear") or a foreign body in the ear should also be considered.

The ear exam is one of the most challenging parts of the pediatric physical examination. You should look at as many normal eardrums as you can to facilitate recognizing the abnormal findings that suggest middle ear infection. A normal eardrum appears smooth, pearly, and translucent, with a sharp light reflex, and the bones of the inner ear are visible through it. An infected eardrum is hyperemic, irregular or bulging in appearance, the light reflex is abnormal or absent, and bony landmarks are obscured. Occasional findings include pus behind the eardrum or fluid in the ear canal, the latter of which suggests a perforated drum or otitis externa.

CASE CONTINUED

VS: Temp 38.9°C (102°F), HR 130, RR 32; Weight 12 kg (80%)

PE: *Gen:* fussy but consolable girl who is crying tears and drinking from her bottle. *HEENT:* mucous membranes are moist and clear, crusting rhinorrhea is noted, pharynx is unremarkable. The left tympanic membrane (TM) is slightly injected, but light reflex and landmarks are clearly visible. The right TM is opaque and red, and has an irregular surface with disturbed light reflex. Bony landmarks are not visualized. Shotty anterior cervical adenopathy is noted, greater on the right than on the left. No nuchal rigidity or photophobia. *Lungs:* clear, no signs of respiratory distress. The remainder of the exam is within normal limits.

THOUGHT QUESTIONS

- What are the most likely causes of this patient's ear infection?
- How will you treat her?

Otitis media is a common childhood infection, accounting for more physician visits than any other pediatric illness. The peak age of incidence is 6 to 36 months. About 30% of cases of acute otitis media are caused by viruses, the other 70% are bacterial in origin. The most common bacterial cause is *Streptococcus pneumoniae* (50%), followed by nontypeable *Haemophilus influenzae* (30%) and *Moraxella catarrhalis* (10% to 15%).

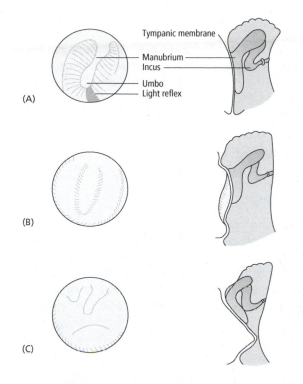

FIGURE 1 Tympanic membrane appearances. **(A)** Normal. **(B)** Otitis media with bulging drum. **(C)** Retracted drum. Used with permission from Rudolf M, Levene M. Paediatrics and Child Health. Oxford: Blackwell Science, Ltd., 1999: 29.

Uncomplicated otitis media is usually treated with a 7 to 10 day course of oral amoxicillin, a safe and inexpensive medication with good coverage against most *S. pneumoniae.* Treatment of recurrent or resistant otitis media may require a change in medications, or preventive measures such as prophylactic antibiotic therapy or ear tubes to vent the middle ear. In many countries otitis media is not routinely treated with antibiotics, because many cases resolve spontaneously.

QUESTIONS

1. All of the following are potential complications of otitis media *except*:
   A. Ear pits
   B. Perforated tympanic membrane
   C. Mastoiditis
   D. Chronic otitis

2. Which of the following is *false* regarding hearing loss from otitis media?
   A. It is the most prevalent complication of otitis media.
   B. It may be associated with high negative pressure in the middle ear.
   C. It is irreversible.
   D. Persistent loss may impair cognitive, language, and emotional development.

3. If this patient had recently (within the last month) been treated with amoxicillin for otitis media, how would you change your management?
   A. Re-treat with amoxicillin, but add Polysporin otic drops
   B. Treat with high-dose amoxicillin or amoxicillin-clavulanic acid
   C. Perform tympanocentesis to identify the organism
   D. Admit for parenteral antibiotic therapy

4. All of the following are risk factors for otitis media *except*:
   A. Breastfeeding
   B. Daycare attendance
   C. Chronic middle ear effusion
   D. Caretaker smoking

ID/CC: 4-year-old boy is brought in by his babysitter for fever and vomiting.

HPI: P.N. developed a fever last night to 103°F, and didn't eat much for dinner. This morning he vomited after breakfast and continued to be febrile, although the fever came down with ibuprofen. Currently he is keeping down some fluids, but has been "lying around" and complaining of a "tummy ache," and the fever has returned. The symptoms have not been accompanied by diarrhea or constipation, cough or upper respiratory infection (URI) symptoms, difficulty breathing, or rash. P.N. has not complained of pain on urination.

PMHx: None   **Meds:** None   **All:** NKDA   **Immunizations:** UTD

SHx: Noncontributory   **FHx:** Noncontributory

VS: Temp 38.9°C (102°F), HR 120, RR 25; Weight 17 kg (50%)

PE: *Gen:* a nontoxic but tired and uncomfortable-appearing boy. *HEENT:* mucous membranes are moist, oropharynx clear, no rhinorrhea, TMs normal. *Abdomen:* diffuse mild tenderness to palpation, without rebound or involuntary guarding. No point tenderness. Normal active bowel sounds. Discomfort on percussion of the back on the left side. *GU:* normal prepubertal male genitalia, uncircumcised penis, testes palpable bilaterally in scrotum without tenderness or redness. No discharge or rashes. *Rectal:* exam is guaiac negative without masses or tenderness, and normal rectal tone. Remainder of exam is within normal limits.

THOUGHT QUESTIONS

- What conditions are in your differential diagnosis at this point for this boy with fever, vomiting, and abdominal pain?
- What laboratory tests or studies would you obtain?

This child presents with fever, vomiting, and abdominal pain, a constellation of symptoms that suggests a wide variety of diagnoses. Briefly, the differential diagnosis should include infectious and noninfectious causes in the abdomen and GU system, as well as infections in other locations such as pneumonia and streptococcal pharyngitis.

Because the abdominal exam does not suggest an acute abdominal process, and the GU and lung exams are normal, studies should be directed toward eliminating the remaining common, treatable causes of fever and abdominal pain, particularly UTI. Specimens of urine may be obtained by catheterizing the bladder, by attaching a bag for collection, or by midstream clean catch of urine, depending on the age of the child. Although a presumptive diagnosis of UTI is often made based on urinalysis results, the gold standard for diagnosis is the urine culture. A specimen should be sent for culture in all cases to identify the organism and its sensitivity.

CASE CONTINUED

A urinalysis is obtained by clean catch midstream with the following results: specific gravity of 1.020, positive blood, positive nitrites, positive leukocyte esterase, otherwise negative. A microscopy of the urine reveals 5–10 RBCs and 50–100 WBCs, as well as positive bacteria. The urine sample is sent for culture.

THOUGHT QUESTIONS

- What does this patient have?
- How would you manage him?

This patient has a UTI. The presence of flank pain and fever suggest pyelonephritis. Urinary tract infections are a common source of fever without localizing signs in infants and children. Although dysuria is an important finding that suggests UTI in older children and adolescents, infants and young children do not typically manifest this symptom, and are more likely to present with fever, poor feeding, vomiting, and abdominal pain.

The bacterial causes of urinary tract infections in children, similar to those in adults, are primarily fecal organisms, the most common being *Escherichia coli*. The goals of treatment of a UTI are to eradicate the infecting organism and to prevent the recurrence and consequences of urinary infections. An uncomplicated UTI or pyelonephritis in the nontoxic child older than 6 months of age is usually treated with a 10- to 14-day course of oral antibiotics; in the toxic or very young child, admission for intravenous therapy is recommended. Follow up should include consideration of imaging to evaluate for anatomic abnormalities or urinary reflux.

QUESTIONS

5. In addition to the proper antibiotic therapy, this patient's management should include:
   A. No further studies
   B. A renal ultrasound
   C. An intravenous pyelogram (IVP)
   D. Prophylactic antibiotics for 1 year

6. All of the following are considered risk factors for UTI *except*:
   A. Female sex
   B. Circumcision
   C. Posterior urethral valve
   D. Recent Foley catheter insertion

7. Typical findings on urinalysis that are consistent with UTI include:
   A. Ketones, glucose, and urobilinogen
   B. Specific gravity greater than 1.025
   C. pH less than 5.0
   D. Positive leukocyte esterase, nitrites, and blood

8. Each of the following are possible consequences of UTI *except*:
   A. Renal scarring
   B. Renal abscess
   C. Ureterocele
   D. Renal failure

ID/CC: 3-month-old infant is brought in by his parents for poor feeding and sleepiness.

HPI: O.B. had been well until yesterday, when he was noted to be sleepier than usual, and today he felt warm to the touch. Although usually a vigorous breastfeeder, he has been taking only small amounts of milk and has vomited once this morning. Today O.B. is difficult to arouse for feeds, and his parents also note that the infant seems to be breathing quickly. The parents deny any history of runny nose, cough, rash, or diarrhea.

PMHx: Unremarkable birth history; no previous illnesses or hospitalizations.

Meds: None   **All:** NKDA   **Immunizations:** UTD

SHx: 4-year-old brother and 6-year-old sister at home; both attend school and are healthy.

FHx: No history of familial metabolic or cardiac disorders, or infant deaths.

VS: Temp 39.2°C (102.5°F), BP 75/40, HR 177 (110–150), RR 48 (25–40); Weight 6.1 kg (50%); O$_2$ saturation 99% on RA.

PE: *Gen:* nontoxic but sleepy, somewhat pale infant who cries when you examine him. *HEENT:* fontanelle is soft but slightly sunken, no rhinorrhea, oropharynx and TMs normal. *Lungs:* tachypneic, lungs clear to auscultation bilaterally, no retractions or grunting. *CV:* tachycardic, no murmur, pulses 2+ throughout, extremities are cool and pink with cap refill approx 3 seconds. *Abdomen:* soft without masses or tenderness. *Skin:* no rashes, jaundice, or petechiae. Remainder of exam is within normal limits.

THOUGHT QUESTIONS
- What possible diagnoses are you most concerned about in this infant?
- What diagnostic workup would you pursue at this time?

This infant has a fever without an apparent source on physical examination. The possibilities for the source of his fever include a viral syndrome, occult bacteremia (defined as a positive blood culture in a well-appearing infant with fever without localizing signs), and a focal bacterial infection not apparent on examination, including UTI, pneumonia, or meningitis.

Due to his young age, his risk for occult bacteremia is about 3% to 5%, and current guidelines recommend laboratory studies to further determine the likelihood of occult or focal bacterial infection. These tests include a complete blood count (CBC), blood culture, urine studies, a chest x-ray in all neonates and in infants with tachypnea or hypoxia, and lumbar puncture in all neonates and in infants in whom meningitis is suggested by history or examination.

This patient's abnormal vital signs, including tachycardia and tachypnea which are important early signs of illness in an infant, may also be due to fever or dehydration. While performing the diagnostic workup, you can correct these conditions and observe the infant for resolution of the vital sign abnormalities.

CASE CONTINUED

A CBC and blood culture are sent, and urine is obtained by catheter for urinalysis and urine culture. While obtaining the blood, you decide to give the infant an intravenous bolus of normal saline (NS), after which he appears pinker, smiles, and begins to breastfeed. Tylenol is given for the fever; with defervescence, the tachycardia and tachypnea resolve. The CBC comes back with a white blood cell (WBC) count of 20,000 with 7% bands, 75% neutrophils, and 15% lymphocytes. The platelets, hemoglobin (Hb) and hematocrit (Hct) are within normal limits. The urinalysis is negative. Blood and urine cultures are pending.

THOUGHT QUESTIONS

- Which laboratory results raise the likelihood for occult bacteremia in this infant?
- How would you manage this infant?

The most concerning laboratory result is the elevated WBC count with left shift (75% neutrophils with bandemia). Febrile infants with a high WBC count are considered at higher risk of occult bacteremia or focal bacterial infection. Based on his young age, well appearance, and high WBC count, current guidelines recommend the empiric treatment of this infant with broad-spectrum antibiotics with close follow up until the final results of all cultures are obtained. A lumbar puncture should be strongly considered prior to starting antibiotics.

CASE CONTINUED

The lumbar puncture shows no signs of meningitis, and a 24-hour dose of ceftriaxone is given. The patient looks great in clinic the next day and gets a second dose of ceftriaxone. On the third day his blood culture grows a few colonies of *Streptococcus pneumoniae*. A repeat blood culture is performed, a third dose of ceftriaxone is given, and the patient is given a 10-day course of oral amoxicillin. The second blood culture and cerebrospinal fluid (CSF) cultures remain negative, and the patient makes a complete recovery.

QUESTIONS

9. The most likely organisms causing occult bacteremia in infants older than 1 month of age are:
    A. *Streptococcus pneumoniae, Haemophilus influenzae* type b, *Neisseria meningitidis*
    B. *S. pneumoniae, Staphylococcus aureus, Staphylococcus epidermidis*
    C. Group B *Streptococcus, Escherichia coli, Listeria monocytogenes*
    D. Group B *Streptococcus, S. aureus, S. epidermidis*

10. Each of the following is considered to increase a febrile child's risk of occult bacteremia *except*:
    A. WBC count >15 or <5
    B. Age <2 years
    C. Temperature >40°C (104°F)
    D. Lower socioeconomic status

11. Sepsis can be differentiated from bacteremia by the presence of:
    A. A high fever
    B. A WBC count greater than 20,000
    C. Hemodynamic instability and/or toxic appearance in the patient
    D. Presence of bacteria in the blood

12. Findings on lumbar puncture that suggest bacterial meningitis include each of the following *except*:
    A. Presence of white blood cells
    B. Presence of red blood cells
    C. Elevated protein
    D. Decreased glucose

ID/CC: 16-year-old girl comes in to the clinic with a lump on her neck.

HPI: M.N. has been feeling sick and tired with a "flu" for about a week. She complains of a fever and a very sore throat, and has been staying home from school. The sore throat makes it difficult to swallow, but she is able to keep down fluids. The lump showed up a few days ago, and is tender. She is otherwise healthy, and no one at home is ill.

PMHx: Unremarkable   **Meds:** Ibuprofen   **All:** NKDA   **Immunizations:** UTD

SHx: Junior in high school, has a boyfriend but is not sexually active; denies drug use; wants to be an engineer. No significant family history.

VS: Temp 39°C (102.2°F), BP 122/80, HR 92, RR 15; Weight 65 kg (80%)

PE: *Gen:* tired-appearing teen, slightly obese, with visible swelling on the left side of her neck. *HEENT:* soft, tender, nonsuppurative 3-cm anterior cervical lymph node palpable on the left. Multiple smaller, tender nodes palpable on the right and left. Oropharynx is remarkable for marked injection with tonsillar exudate. There is no nuchal rigidity, photophobia, or sinus tenderness, and no further lymphadenopathy is noted on exam. *Abdomen:* soft, spleen tip is palpable and slightly tender on the left, no hepatomegaly. Remainder of exam is within normal limits.

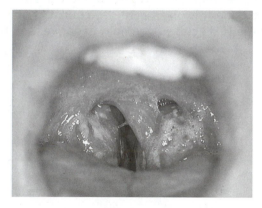

FIGURE 4 Exudative tonsillitis, as might be seen on this patient. Used with permission from Rudolf M, Levene M. Paediatrics and Child Health. Oxford: Blackwell Science, Ltd., 1999: 104.

THOUGHT QUESTIONS

- What is your differential diagnosis at this point?
- What laboratory tests or studies would you consider to help with your diagnosis?

This patient is a teen with an enlarged and tender cervical lymph node, as well as bilateral cervical lymphadenopathy and signs of upper respiratory illness. Cervical adenopathy is a common and usually benign finding in children, as the cervical nodes enlarge in reaction to many viral illnesses. However, asymmetric, hard, painful, or generalized adenopathy deserves further investigation, as the cause may be an infection in the node itself or a serious systemic illness. Most acute lymphadenopathy is infectious in origin. The most common causes are viruses, particularly Epstein-Barr virus (EBV), cytomegalovirus (CMV), adenovirus, and human immunodeficiency virus (HIV). Subacute or chronic lymphadenopathy is also likely to be infectious in origin. However, noninfectious causes of adenopathy, such as malignancy and congenital neck masses, should be strongly considered in cases of chronic lymphadenopathy.

In considering the differential diagnoses it is important to take into account the age of the child, the acute versus chronic nature of the adenopathy, and whether it is local or generalized. Associated findings such as rash, hepatosplenomegaly, and a history of recent illness or weight loss are also important to elicit. Laboratory tests and studies should be guided by the patient's presentation, and the suspicion of an infectious or noninfectious cause. This teen has symptoms suggestive of an acute viral illness, in particular acute mononucleosis. Other viral infections, bacterial adenitis, group A *Streptococcus* (GAS) pharyngitis, and malignancy should also be considered. A CBC is a good initial screening tool for this broad differential, as it will identify signs of inflammation and basic immune function, both helpful in this case. More specific diagnostic tests include the Monospot, a heterophile antibody test for EBV infection that is available in most centers, and a rapid test for GAS.

CASE CONTINUED

Labs: CBC reveals WBC of 20 with 15% atypical lymphs, Hct of 38, platelets of 175. A Monospot is positive for heterophile antibodies to EBV. Rapid Strep screen negative.

THOUGHT QUESTIONS

• What does this patient have?
• How will you manage her?

This patient's clinical picture and laboratory results support a diagnosis of acute mononucleosis syndrome, usually caused by infection with EBV. Although EBV acquired in early childhood usually causes a subclinical picture, infection in adolescence or adulthood results in the classic mononucleosis syndrome of fever, exudative pharyngitis, and lymphadenopathy. Profound malaise and fatigue often accompany the syndrome, and may last for weeks to months. Treatment of mononucleosis is generally supportive, consisting of pain and fever control. In this patient, who has an enlarged and tender spleen, avoidance of contact sports should be advised until the spleen is back to normal.

QUESTIONS

13. Complications of EBV infection include all of the following *except*:
    A. Splenic rupture
    B. Neutropenia
    C. Brain abscess
    D. Airway obstruction

14. Diagnosis of mononucleosis is usually made by:
    A. Clinical criteria, supported by laboratory findings
    B. Throat culture for EBV
    C. Lymph node biopsy
    D. The presence of an enlarged spleen on examination

15. In a 2-year-old child with suppurative adenitis, what is the most likely cause?
    A. Tuberculosis
    B. *Staphylococcus aureus* infection
    C. Anaerobic organisms
    D. Catscratch disease

16. Which of the following is *not* a likely cause of subacute or chronic lymphadenopathy in children?
    A. Acute lymphocytic leukemia
    B. Strep throat
    C. Catscratch disease
    D. Tuberculosis

ID/CC: 15-month-old girl is brought in by her mother for a fever and refusal to drink.

HPI: H.D. was well until last night, when she felt hot to the touch, and refused her bottle. After some Tylenol she seemed better. Mother also noticed "spots" on her hands and a diaper rash. Since this morning H.D. has been pushing away her bottle and has been fussy. Mother measured her temperature at 104°F rectally and gave her a half dose of Tylenol. She brought the child in because she was concerned about giving so much medicine.

PMHx: Normal birth history, no prior hospitalizations or serious illnesses.

Meds: Tylenol for fever   **All:** NKDA   **Immunizations:** UTD to 1 year

SHx: Lives with single mother, attends daycare; 6-year-old brother has asthma. No current sick contacts at home.

FHx: Noncontributory.

THOUGHT QUESTIONS

- What will you look for on the examination of this patient?
- How can you evaluate her hydration status, as she has not been drinking well?

This child appears well but has a high fever, so you must either establish an identifiable viral or bacterial source for the fever, or begin a workup for occult infection or bacteremia. Many viral syndromes include classic but subtle findings hidden in the mouth or on the skin (including palms and soles), so your search for a fever source should include careful examination of these areas as well as the ears, throat, and lungs.

Assessment of hydration status includes a thorough history of fluid intake and urine and stool output, as well as an assessment of mucous membranes, tear production, skin turgor and perfusion, and cardiovascular stability. A child under 10 kg should take in at least 60 cc/kg per day (2 oz/kg per day) and urinate a minimum of three times in a 24-hour period. Intake or output below these minimums should raise concern for dehydration.

CASE CONTINUED

H.D. has urinated twice since this morning, and she has had one normal stool. Her total intake since the fever started has been two 8-oz bottles of milk and 4 oz of juice, but no solids.

VS: Temp 38.9°C (102°F), HR 140, RR 30; Weight 9 kg (80%)

PE: *Gen:* fussy but consolable girl, drooling and occasionally mouthing her bottle, then pushing it away. *HEENT:* TMs clear bilaterally, crying tears, moist mucous membranes. The oropharynx is remarkable for several shallow grayish vesicles on posterior oropharynx, and one on the base of the tongue. There are no lip lesions. *Lungs:* CTAB, no stridor, grunting, flaring, or retracting. *Skin:* capillary refill is brisk, <3 seconds, and the skin is well perfused. Careful examination of hands and feet reveals several shallow, linear gray vesicles on the fingers of both hands, and one on the left sole. The perineum is remarkable for a diffuse mildly erythematous maculopapular rash.

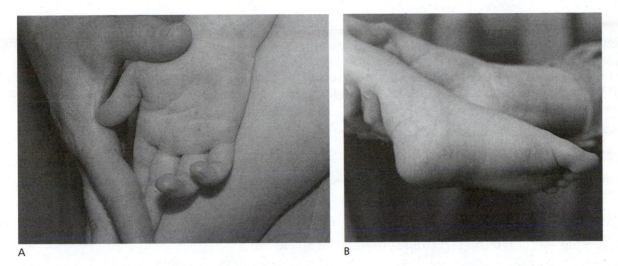

A   B

FIGURE 5 (A, B) Appearance of lesions on this patient's extremities. Used with permission from Banniser B, Begg N, Gillespie S. Infectious Disease, 2nd ed. Oxford: Blackwell Science, Ltd., 2000: plate 5.10.

THOUGHT QUESTIONS

- What is your differential diagnosis, and most likely diagnosis?
- What is the most likely morbidity from this condition, and how will you manage it?

The differential diagnosis in this case should include several common viral illnesses associated with rash and/or oral findings, including parvovirus (fifth disease), human herpesvirus 6 (HHV-6, roseola), herpes simplex virus (HSV), measles, and varicella. Nonviral illnesses in the differential diagnosis include Kawasaki syndrome and toxic shock syndrome. This patient, however, has the classic findings of infection by coxsackie virus A, otherwise known as hand-foot-and-mouth disease.

Most prevalent in the spring and summer, this common virus causes a prodrome of high fever, anorexia, and oral pain ("herpangina"). Typical skin and oral findings follow, which include painful, shallow, linear grayish or whitish vesicles on the posterior oropharynx and posterior third of the tongue, and similar but usually painless lesions on the palms and soles. The presentation may include some or all of these findings. The diagnosis of this infection is clinical, and can be easily missed without a thorough physical examination. The primary morbidity from hand-foot-and-mouth disease is dehydration. Pain is often severe, and young children may refuse to drink for days at a time. To avoid dehydration, pain and fever control are essential.

QUESTIONS

17. Each of the following are indicated in the management of this patient *except*:
    A. Oral and/or topical pain medications
    B. Antipyretics
    C. Careful observation for dehydration
    D. Antivirals

18. Which of the following viral exanthems is characterized by a "slapped-cheek" rash?
    A. Measles
    B. Rubella
    C. Roseola (sixth disease)
    D. Parvovirus (fifth disease)

19. Treatment of varicella (chickenpox) with acyclovir is generally *not* indicated in which group of children?
    A. Newborns
    B. Teenagers
    C. Immunocompromised children
    D. Toddlers

20. Kawasaki disease is characterized by fever, rash, and all of the following *except*:
    A. Nonpurulent conjunctivitis
    B. Erythema of palms and soles
    C. Vomiting
    D. Acute unilateral cervical adenopathy

ID/CC: 6-month-old girl is brought in to the clinic for fever and crying since this morning.

HPI: B.M., who had been previously healthy, vomited after feeding this morning and since then has been inconsolable. She refused feeds the rest of the day, vomited twice more, and has been crying "as if something is hurting her." Just before taking her to the clinic, her mother noticed that her face felt hot, but that her hands and feet were cool. She has had a cold for a couple of days, but has been otherwise well.

PMHx: Normal birth history, no complications, no illness or hospitalizations.

Meds: None   **All:** NKDA

Immunizations: Parents have elected not to immunize their three children, who have "always been healthy."

SHx: 3-year-old brother had an ear infection recently; otherwise, the family is healthy.

VS: Temp 40.1°C (104.1°F), HR 180 (110–130), RR 56 (30–40)

PE: *Gen:* lethargic female infant who becomes very irritable with a shrill cry whenever she is touched or moved, and is not consolable. *HEENT:* anterior fontanelle bulging and firm, mucus membranes slightly dry, oropharynx clear, no lymphadenopathy. *Lungs:* tachypneic, lungs are clear. *CV:* tachycardic, extremities cool, with cap refill 3 to 4 seconds. *Skin:* no rashes or petechiae.

THOUGHT QUESTIONS

- What diagnosis are you most concerned about in this infant?
- What further workup would you like to obtain?

In this febrile, irritable, and toxic-appearing infant you should be most concerned about meningitis, sepsis, or another serious invasive bacterial infection. Although nuchal rigidity is an important finding that suggests meningitis in older children, it is generally not found in infants less than 1 year of age who have an open fontanelle. Other conditions in the differential diagnoses include nonbacterial (aseptic) meningitis and other conditions causing increased ICP, such as an intracranial hemorrhage, abscess, or mass.

As in any toxic infant, your first concern should be the ABCs (airway, breathing, and circulation). Thus, measures should be taken immediately to ensure adequate ventilation and hemodynamic stability. Further workup and administration of antibiotics should occur in a timely fashion following stabilization of the patient. Because you are primarily concerned about infection, a CBC and cultures of blood, urine, and CSF should be obtained, preferably before the administration of antibiotics.

CASE CONTINUED

You obtain IV access quickly and begin a bolus of normal saline (NS). You draw a CBC and blood culture, obtain urine by catheter, and perform a lumbar puncture. Immediately after obtaining all cultures, you give the patient a dose of IV ceftriaxone and vancomycin for broad-spectrum coverage against gram-positive and gram-negative organisms. Soon afterward, the lab calls with the results of the lumbar puncture: the WBC count is 700, red blood cell (RBC) count is 2, with a total protein of 150 (50–80) and glucose of 25 (>50). Gram-positive diplococci are seen on gram stain of the CSF.

> **THOUGHT QUESTIONS**
> * What does this patient have?
> * How will you manage her?

This patient has acute bacterial meningitis, presumably caused by *Streptococcus pneumoniae*, based on the gram stain results. This dangerous infection, with a mortality of 1% to 8% after the neonatal period, occurs when bacteria gain access to the CSF. Risk factors for meningitis include otitis media, sinusitis, CSF leak (e.g., from skull fracture), and immunodeficiency (e.g., sickle cell disease, AIDS). The prognosis with early diagnosis and treatment is good, but as many as 50% of patients will have some neurodevelopmental sequelae. A vaccine against seven common serotypes of *S. pneumoniae* is now part of the routine vaccination schedule, and is expected to reduce the incidence of meningitis.

Patients with acute bacterial meningitis should be hospitalized for IV antibiotic therapy and observation for increased intracranial pressure, seizures, or other neurologic sequelae. Audiologic testing should be performed prior to discharge and on follow-up evaluations. For meningitis caused by *Haemophilus influenzae* or *Neisseria meningitidis*, prophylaxis of family members and close contacts is indicated.

QUESTIONS

21. The most common causes of bacterial meningitis in children over 1 month of age are:
    A. *S. pneumoniae, N. meningitidis*, and *H. influenzae*
    B. *E. coli*, group B *Streptococcus*, and *Listeria*
    C. *S. pneumoniae*, nontypeable *H. influenzae*, and *Moraxella catarrhalis*
    D. *S. pneumoniae, S. aureus*, and *Pseudomonas aeruginosa*

22. The most common sequela of meningitis in children is:
    A. Sensorineural hearing loss
    B. Mental retardation
    C. Seizures
    D. Behavioral problems
    E. Paralysis

23. Which of the following findings on lumbar puncture suggests bacterial meningitis?
    A. Numerous red blood cells
    B. Low protein
    C. Low glucose
    D. Lymphocyte predominance

24. The primary cause of aseptic (nonbacterial) meningitis in children is:
    A. Varicella (VZV)
    B. *Cryptococcus*
    C. Enterovirus
    D. Herpes simplex virus (HSV)
    E. Mumps

ID/CC: 15-month-old boy with cough and difficulty breathing is brought in by his mother.

HPI: H.I. presents with a 4-day history of rhinorrhea, low-grade fever, and mild cough. His mother states that the cough has progressively become worse over the last 36 hours and now sounds "terrible." His mother was concerned that he was having difficulty catching his breath and was breathing very fast, and she subsequently brought him to see you. He has refused to eat or drink today. The mother states that he attends daycare and "one of the older children may have a throat infection."

PMHx: SVD at term with no complications, no hospitalizations, no chronic illnesses.

Meds: Over-the-counter decongestant/cough suppressant, acetaminophen   **All:** NKDA

Immunizations: Received 2, 4, 6, and 12 month vaccines.

SHx: Lives with parents; no smokers, no pets in household.

DevHx: *ROS:* As above, no vomiting or diarrhea, no rash.

VS: Temp 100.3°F, BP 100/55, HR 130, RR 42, pulse oximetry 97% on room air, decreases to 90% during coughing episode

PE: *Gen:* alert, nontoxic appearing, comfortable while supine in mother's lap but crying as you approach, with audible hoarseness and inspiratory stridor, and a "barking" cough. *HEENT:* mild nasal flaring with inspiration, TMs erythematous but otherwise clear. Oropharynx erythematous with no exudate, mucosa moist. *Lungs:* sternal and mild supraclavicular retractions, no crackles, rhonchi audible in middle fields, no audible wheezing. *CV:* RR&R, no murmur, capillary refill time <2 seconds, strong pulses throughout.

THOUGHT QUESTIONS

- What is in this patient's differential diagnosis?
- What components of this history and physical should help in your diagnosis?
- What additional studies may aid in making a diagnosis?

The differential diagnosis for this patient includes the various causes of upper airway obstruction in this age group. This includes acute laryngotracheitis (croup), epiglottitis, pneumonia, foreign body aspiration, bacterial tracheitis, underlying laryngotracheomalacia, retropharyngeal or peritonsillar abscess, or ingestion of caustic agents. Previous history of intubation may lead to inclusion of sub-glottic stenosis.

On history and physical examination, the course of presentation, with mild but progressive upper respiratory tract symptoms, characteristic "barking" seal-like cough, and inspiratory stridor are all suggestive of croup. The initial visual evaluation of the child's appearance, along with the physical examination, illustrates the most frequent serious diagnostic problem in helping to distinguish croup from epiglottitis. The patient is comfortable while supine, nontoxic appearing, and not distressed or with apprehension, all of which may help lessen the likelihood of epiglottitis.

Traditionally, croup is a clinical diagnosis, but some tools can be used to support your initial findings. Lateral plain films of the neck may reveal narrowing of the air column in the subglottic area, known as the "steeple" sign. The CBC may reveal leukocytosis. Pulse oximetry is generally normal, but may be decreased during coughing episodes and with superimposed lower airway involvement.

CASE CONTINUED

The patient is initially treated with cool mist aerosol while sitting on his parent's lap. After initially responding with decreased stridor and cough, his symptoms return and he develops an audible wheeze with slightly worse retractions. His pulse oximetry is 97% on room air.

QUESTIONS

25. At this time, the next likely step in management should be:
    A. A trial of nebulized albuterol
    B. A trial of nebulized racemic epinephrine
    C. Endoscopic evaluation of the child's airway in a controlled setting
    D. Intravenous antibiotics
    E. More cool mist and comfort

26. The likely organism involved in this disease process is:
    A. *Haemophilus influenzae*
    B. Respiratory syncytial virus (RSV)
    C. *Streptococcus pneumoniae*
    D. Parainfluenza virus species
    E. Epstein-Barr virus

27. Which of the following statements about croup are *true*?
    A. Most children with croup are symptomatic enough to prompt medical attention.
    B. The best way to distinguish croup from epiglottitis is via direct laryngoscopy in the operating room.
    C. Croup generally is a lower airway disease, and wheezing is commonly found.
    D. Croup affects only younger children.

28. Which of the following statements regarding epiglottitis are *true*?
    A. Fever, sore throat, stridor, and drooling are common upon presentation.
    B. Lateral neck films may show a "thumbprint" sign, but are not recommended given the delay in therapy.
    C. Epiglottitis is an acute airway emergency.
    D. The incidence has decreased due to routine *H. influenzae* type B vaccination.
    E. All of the above.

ID/CC: 2-year-old boy with a 2-day history of cough and "noisy"/difficult breathing.

HPI: F.B. was previously well, but his father noticed yesterday that he had "noisy" breathing. He seemed to have some difficulty, which was temporarily relieved by steam mist. Today, he has been coughing and has some audible wheezing. He has no fever or runny nose. He has not had any vomiting or diarrhea, nor has he had any rash. The child has refused feeding today and has been less active. His father says he was worried because he noticed a faster rate of breathing and that the child was having more difficulty breathing. He tried administering albuterol from a previous prescription, without any success.

PMHx: Hospitalized for bronchiolitis at 6 months of age, born at term without complications.

Meds: Albuterol as above   **All:** NKDA

SHx: Lives with father and 5-year-old sibling.

VS: Temp 99.5°F, HR 135, RR 45; Pulse oximetry: 88% on room air.

PE: *Gen:* sitting in father's lap, tachypneic, visible intercostal retractions, appears in moderate respiratory distress. *HEENT:* oropharynx is slightly erythematous, but otherwise clear. *Lungs:* intermittent mild coughing, decreased expiratory breath sounds on right side, with mild inspiratory stridor, with expiratory wheezes at bases R>L, fine crackles heard at right base. Rest of exam is within normal limits.

THOUGHT QUESTIONS

- What is in the differential diagnosis?
- What additional history may be helpful in this case?
- What diagnostic/therapeutic evaluations are indicated for this child?

The differential diagnosis in this case includes asthma, pneumonia, foreign body aspiration, and other causes of obstructive airway disease. Although the age and possibility of aspirating a small object or the toy of a nearby toddler are suggestive on their own, it is unlikely that a given history of observed aspiration of a foreign body will lead to the diagnosis. Signs and symptoms of acute onset of inspiratory stridor, unilateral ausculatory findings, and chest x-ray findings all suggest the diagnosis of foreign body aspiration. Due to its course and natural continuity with the upper airways, the right mainstem bronchus is the most common site for foreign bodies to be found. A chest x-ray that reveals hyperinflation of one lung (usually the right), which persists during films obtained during expiration and in the right lateral decubitus position, suggests a possible "ball valve" mechanism of obstruction secondary to a likely partial foreign body obstruction. If a foreign body aspiration is suspected, the definitive diagnosis is made with bronchoscopy, which can also be used to remove the foreign object.

CASE CONTINUED

A chest x-ray is obtained, which reveals hyperinflation of the right lung. F.B. is admitted to the hospital for rigid bronchoscopy. During the procedure a peanut is discovered and removed from the right mainstem bronchus. After the procedure, the child is discharged to home after a discussion of aspiration precautions with his parents.

QUESTIONS

29. Which of the following is *not* usually an early sign or symptom related to foreign body aspiration?
    A. Retractions
    B. Stridor
    C. Wheezing
    D. Cough
    E. Blood-tinged sputum

30. What is the most likely age at presentation for a foreign body aspiration?
    A. 6 to 36 months
    B. 4 to 5 years
    C. 0 to 6 months
    D. 6 to 11 years
    E. 11 to 15 years

31. Expiratory chest x-ray in a complete right mainstem bronchus obstruction should demonstrate:
    A. Left lung hyperinflation with mediastinal shift toward right
    B. Left lung atelectasis with heart drawn to left side
    C. Right lung atelectasis with heart drawn to right side
    D. Right lung hyperinflation with mediastinal shift toward left

32. Which of the following statements are *false*?
    A. Foreign body aspiration into the trachea is more common than the lower airway.
    B. Nuts account for over 50% of foreign body aspiration.
    C. Patients may present up to a week after initial event of choking.
    D. Most patients recover quickly after removal with minimal sequelae.

ID/CC: 2 1/2-year-old girl with 2 days of cough, runny nose, vomiting, and irritability.

HPI: B.P. is brought into the emergency room after having had a cough, vomiting, and diarrhea for nearly 2 days. The parents note that she had started having a runny nose and fever 2 days ago. She subsequently began vomiting a clear, nonbilious fluid and her stools were loose. The child's fever was treated with acetaminophen. She has not been active and today has been increasingly irritable, refusing any oral intake. She has a wet cough; it has not seemed to respond to over-the-counter antitussive medicines. Both parents are concerned that the child seems "like she's losing too much fluid" and "doesn't seem like herself." They also state that "everyone is sick at daycare."

PMHx: Normal birth history, no previous hospitalizations.

Meds: Tylenol as above   **All:** NKDA   **Immunizations:** UTD to 2 years

SHx: Lives with mother and father, attends daycare; mother expecting second child.

FHx: Noncontributory.

VS: Temp 102.5°F, HR 150, RR 25

PE: *Gen:* child lies quietly on mother's lap, not appearing in any acute distress. *HEENT:* mild rhinorrhea, somewhat dry oral mucosa, otherwise normal. *Neck:* supple. *Chest:* decreased breath sounds at bases, no crackles or wheezes. *CV:* tachycardic, otherwise normal exam. *Abdomen:* tenderness on right side on deep palpation, otherwise normal. *Skin:* turgor is slightly decreased. Remainder of exam within normal limits.

THOUGHT QUESTIONS

- What is in this patient's differential diagnosis?
- What diagnostic studies would you like performed?

The differential diagnosis for this patient includes gastroenteritis and other intra-abdominal processes. In addition, accompanying upper respiratory tract symptoms and rash would usually suggest a systemic viral illness. Included in the differential diagnosis should be urinary tract infections and pneumonia, due to the age of the patient and the presence of systemic constitutional complaints. In patients who present with these symptoms, common laboratory tests that are obtained include a CBC, blood culture, liver function tests, and serum electrolytes. Because of her abdominal symptoms, a kidney and upper bladder (KUB) and upright would be recommended; the URI symptoms might lead to obtaining a chest x-ray.

CASE CONTINUED

On admission to the hospital, a blood culture was obtained, as were a CBC, transaminases, bilirubins, and serum electrolytes. Of note, her serum HCO_3 level was found to be 14, and her WBC was 25,000 (66% neutrophils, and 19% bands). Urinalysis revealed no abnormalities. A plain film of the abdomen was essentially normal. After several hours, the child had persistent cough and vomiting, was now in more discomfort, and seemed to be somewhat tachypneic. A chest x-ray revealed a consolidation of her right lower lobe with a small pleural effusion, suggesting a bacterial pneumonia. The patient was treated with the appropriate antibiotics and discharged home after an uncomplicated hospital course.

QUESTIONS

33. For the above patient, what is the most common cause of bacterial pneumonia?
    A. *Mycoplasma pneumoniae*
    B. Group B streptococci
    C. *Chlamydia pneumoniae*
    D. *Streptococcus pneumoniae*
    E. *Haemophilus influenzae* type B

34. Which of the following conditions is associated with an increased risk of bacterial pneumonia?
    A. Bronchopulmonary dysplasia
    B. Cystic fibrosis
    C. Gastroesophageal reflux/aspiration
    D. Sickle cell disease
    E. All of the above

35. When assessing the older child or adolescent with suspected pneumonia, which of the medications listed is useful against *Mycoplasma pneumoniae* infection?
    A. Ribavirin
    B. Penicillin
    C. Amoxicillin
    D. Amoxicillin-clavulanic acid
    E. Erythromycin

36. Which of the following statements are *true*?
    A. Tachypnea and chest discomfort are the most common indications of pneumonia.
    B. Up to 50% of patients with bacterial pneumonia show concurrent viral disease.
    C. For outpatients, amoxicillin is sufficient for most cases of bacterial pneumonia.
    D. Infants with bacterial pneumonia may present with nonspecific symptoms.
    E. All of the above.

ID/CC: 6-year-old girl with cough for 3 weeks.

HPI: A.E. was well until 3 weeks ago, when she developed cough, rhinorrhea, sore throat, and low-grade fever. She refused to play outside at that time stating that she "was out of breath from coughing." Her rhinorrhea, sore throat, and fever resolved, but the cough has persisted. Mother states that it is worse at night, and although she is active, "she still gets tired when she plays." She gets occasional headaches, has no current nausea, vomiting, or diarrhea. She has no rashes currently. Mother has tried several over-the-counter cough remedies without success. She states that she thinks it is a lingering "cold" and that "they seem to take longer to clear," as they did for her at that age.

PMHx: None; normal birth history with no complications.

Meds: As above   **All:** NKDA

SHx: Lives with mother and father; mother smokes "outside the house"; pets: one cat.

FHx: Mother has "recurrent bronchitis attacks."

VS: Temp 98.8°F, BP 95/55, HR 100, RR 20

PE: *Gen:* well-appearing girl in no apparent distress, with intermittent cough during exam. *HEENT:* oropharynx slightly erythematous, TMs within normal limits, no intranasal lesions. *Lungs:* decreased breath sounds at bases bilaterally, with rhonchi throughout fields, increased expiratory phase, with wheezing in middle lung fields (medial>lateral), no crackles. *CV:* RR&R, normal S_1, S_2, no murmur. *Ext:* no clubbing, no cyanosis, no edema.

THOUGHT QUESTIONS

- What is in the differential diagnosis at this point?
- What bedside maneuvers can help in narrowing the diagnosis?
- What laboratory or imaging studies may be useful for this patient?
- What further history would you obtain?

The differential diagnosis for chronic cough is extensive and includes reactive airway disease (RAD: asthma), gastroesophageal reflux disease (GERD), aspirated foreign body, sinusitis, and allergies. Less likely in face of an otherwise normal history and physical examination would be causes of immune deficiency, cystic fibrosis, ciliary or parenchymal abnormalities, and psychogenic causes. In this case, a peak flow measurement was obtained and was found to be 50% of the expected value for her height, indicating an obstructive airway process. Laboratory tests were not performed and a chest x-ray revealed hyperinflation and several areas of likely atelectasis at the bases bilaterally. Given the above findings and history (night-time cough, cough with exercise), the diagnosis of asthma was made.

A thorough history should be obtained for every patient with a suspicion of asthma. This should include a detailed history of the cough, medications, precipitating factors, ill contacts, travel, pets, environmental factors at home and school, family history, and a review of systems.

Although asthma is generally a clinical diagnosis that is reversible with bronchodilators and anti-inflammatory agents, some laboratory testing may be useful to distinguish between other causes of chronic cough. This would possibly include a CBC (eosinophilia may suggest asthma/atopy), sputum samples for gram stain and culture, and immunologic studies. A purified protein derivative (PPD) test should be placed for suspicion of tuberculosis. Further imaging and studies should be guided by your history and physical examination.

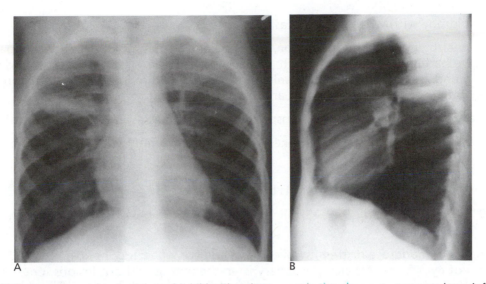

FIGURE 10 (A, B) These radiographs of a 3-year-old child with asthma exacerbation demonstrate severe hyperinflation, increased anteroposterior diameter of the chest, and several areas of atelectasis. Used with permission from Marino B, Snead K, McMillan J. Blueprints in Pediatrics, 2nd ed. Malden: Blackwell Science, Inc., 2001: 275.

CASE CONTINUED

After a nebulized β-agonist bronchodilator treatment, the patient's peak flow improved and she was sent home on β-agonist and cromolyn sodium metered-dose inhaler therapy. She returned 6 weeks later to the emergency department in respiratory distress with shortness of breath, tachypnea (RR 50), audible wheezing, subcostal retractions, and supraclavicular retractions. Her pulse oximetry reading was 88% on room air. The lung examination revealed decreased breath sounds and no wheezing in all fields. Blood gas analysis revealed a pH of 7.48 , a $PaCO_2$ of 28, a PaO_2 of 65, and a base deficit of –2. She had not been taking her medications for several weeks, as she had improved and her parents felt she did not need any further therapy.

QUESTIONS

37. Based on this description, which of the following would now be an appropriate course of initial therapy?
    A. Cromolyn sodium
    B. Oxygen and leukotriene receptor agonists
    C. Oxygen and inhaled bronchodilators
    D. IV fluids
    E. Oxygen, inhaled bronchodilators, and systemic corticosteroids

38. Which is generally *not* considered a component of reactive airway disease?
    A. Bronchospasm
    B. Mucus secretion
    C. Inflammation surrounding the airway
    D. Irreversible airway obstruction

39. Which of the following is a *true* statement about asthma?
    A. In acute asthma, blood gas analysis revealing a low $PaCO_2$ suggests a respiratory alkalosis compensation for a primary metabolic acidosis process.
    B. Asthma triggers may be cold temperature, infections, exercise, anxiety, and smoke exposure.
    C. In acute asthma, decreased breath sounds but no wheezing is a sign of improvement.
    D. Aside from nebulized bronchodilators, there are no other medications available for immediate relief of airway constriction.
    E. Mortality has declined in recent years due primarily to advances in therapy.

40. Which of the following are risk factors for reactive airway disease?
    A. Atopy
    B. Genetic predisposition
    C. Smoke exposure
    D. Urban households
    E. All of the above

ID/CC: 5-year-old boy with wheezing and rash presents to the emergency room.

HPI: A.R. was healthy prior to this afternoon, when he and his parents were at a local park for a birthday party. He had been seen playing with some other children, when he was noticed to have difficulty breathing and was wheezing, with swelling of his face, and redness of his face and neck. His voice sounds a "little hoarse" to his parents, and he is crying.

PMHx: Normal birth history, no previous hospitalizations or illnesses, history of mild asthma.

PSHx: None   **Meds:** β-Agonist inhaler taken as needed, takes multivitamin supplement

All: NKDA

SHx: Lives with parents, no siblings, no pets because of allergies.

VS: Temp 99°F, BP 82/40 (systolic 80–125) HR 145 (90–110), RR 35 (18–25); Pulse oximetry: 88% on room air.

PE: *Gen:* appears in moderate distress, swollen face, audible wheezing, hoarse voice. *HEENT:* erythematous swelling of eyes/face, TMs clear, oropharynx erythematous without lesions. *Chest:* visible suprasternal and intercostal retractions, wheezing in all fields with adequate air entry, no crackles. *CV:* RR&R tachycardic, no murmur, capillary refill time <3 seconds. *Skin:* erythematous, raised, circumscribed, edematous white/evanescent plaques on face, neck, and upper extremities/trunk. *Neuro:* gross nonfocal. Rest of exam is within normal limits.

THOUGHT QUESTIONS

- What further history would you like to obtain?
- What is in your differential diagnosis at this point?
- What are your immediate concerns regarding this patient?

This child shows all of the signs and symptoms of an anaphylactic reaction. Further history from the parents reveals that the boy had been stung by a bee. The most common causes of anaphylactic reactions in children include *Hymenoptera* stings (bees and wasps); drugs such as penicillin and local anesthetics, foods such as peanuts, eggs, and seafood; and blood products, contrast media, and latex. Obtaining a history of events leading up to the episode may help determine exposure to the antigen. Also, obtaining a thorough past history indicative of underlying disorders may give clues to the cause and the clinical presentation. Previous asthma may be a risk factor for bronchospasm during anaphylactic reactions. Underlying spina bifida or urologic disorders may predispose an individual to latex allergies.

The differential diagnosis for systemic anaphylaxis includes seizures, arrhythmias, syncopal episodes, foreign body aspiration, acute poisoning, or ingestion/inhalation.

Anaphylaxis is an extreme systemic allergic reaction, is a type 1 hypersensitivity reaction, and can be characterized by cutaneous, respiratory, cardiovascular, and gastrointestinal features. The physical exam should initially focus on vital signs and ABC: airway, breathing, and circulation. In this patient, his vitals and examination were indicative of airway swelling and bronchospasm, urticaria and angioedema, tachycardia, and borderline hypotension. With ingested allergens, diarrhea and abdominal pain may accompany presentation, likely due to angioedema within the gastrointestinal (GI) tract.

Urticaria and angioedema are common manifestations of anaphylaxis as well as other allergic reactions in children. They involve exposure to the above-mentioned allergens as well as hereditary forms. Children with known reactions to specific allergens such as bee stings should always be advised to carry injectable epinephrine to minimize future attacks.

CASE CONTINUED

You treat A.R. appropriately and discuss precautions to take in the future with his parents. Within a short time his symptoms have diminished and he is discharged to home.

QUESTIONS

41. Which of the following statements are true about anaphylactic reactions?
    A. An IgM-mediated reaction that occurs several days after allergen exposure
    B. An IgE-mediated reaction that occurs several days after allergen exposure
    C. An IgM-mediated reaction that occurs several hours after allergen exposure
    D. An IgE- and histamine-mediated reaction that occurs hours after allergen exposure

42. Which of the following are *not* typical characteristics of urticaria?
    A. Pruritic
    B. Generally resolve within 24 hours
    C. Nonblanching lesions
    D. Results from vascular dilatation and increased permeability

43. Which of the following are *not* typical characteristics of angioedema?
    A. Confined to the epidermis
    B. Nonpruritic
    C. Well-demarcated areas of swelling
    D. Generally resolves within a few hours to days

44. Which of the following is indicated in the initial treatment of anaphylaxis?
    A. Airway support, oxygen, and IV fluids
    B. Subcutaneous epinephrine
    C. Diphenhydramine
    D. Corticosteroids
    E. All of the above

ID/CC: 6-month-old girl with fever, cough, and rapid breathing.

HPI: R.B. presents to your winter evening clinic with a 4-day history of fever, rhinorrhea, and cough which has worsened. Since last night, she has had a progressively increasing rate of breathing and worsening symptoms. Her mother reports that, during that time, she has become more irritable and is having a harder time breathing. She had been tolerating her feeds well until today, and now is refusing her bottle. She has had no vomiting or diarrhea. She attends daycare, where there are numerous ill contacts.

PMHx: None. *Birth:* SVD at term without complications.

PSHx: None   **Meds:** Acetaminophen as needed for fever

All: NKDA   **Immunizations:** UTD

DietHx: Just started solids last week, bottle feeding on formula.

DevHx: Sits without support, babbling, transferring objects. *ROS:* no rash, no wet diapers since this morning.

SHx: Lives with mother and grandmother at home; smokers in home.

FHx: Father with reactive airway disease.

VS: Temp 101°F, BP 95/55, HR 165, RR 58; Weight: 6.5 kg (50th percentile)

PE: *Gen:* alert, interactive, crying infant, grunting mildly with each breath. *HEENT:* normocephalic and atraumatic (NCAT), AFO to 1 cm, pupils equal, round, reactive to light and accommodation (PERRLA), copious nasal secretions, nasal flaring. Oropharynx erythematous, TMs with erythema/no exudates/good landmarks. *Chest:* intercostal retractions, shallow rapid breathing, wheezing audible in all fields, decreased aeration at bases, some crackles heard at bases. *CV:* RR&R tachycardic, normal S_1, S_2, no murmur, cap refill is 2.5 seconds and pulses normal. *Abdomen:* distended but soft, positive bowel sounds, no visceromegaly, nontender. *Neuro:* grossly nonfocal. *Skin:* no lesions.

THOUGHT QUESTIONS

- What are some initial evaluations/therapeutic measures that can be taken for this patient?
- What is the differential diagnosis for this patient?
- What diagnostic tests may aid in making this diagnosis?

For the infant in respiratory distress (which is usually signified by grunting, flaring of the nostrils, and retractions/use of accessory respiratory muscles), one must always be aware of the ABCs: airway, breathing, and circulation. Once hemodynamic stability and a patent airway with breathing is established, assessing the patient's oxygen saturation may be the next step. Oxygen is a natural bronchodilator and can help this type of patient. Fluid support may also be warranted. The differential diagnosis for this patient would include bronchiolitis, pneumonia, reactive airway disease, and aspiration of foreign body. Clinical examination and history are generally sufficient to initially manage the patient; however, some tests such as viral antigen assays and chest x-rays may aid in making the diagnosis.

CASE CONTINUED

Pulse oximetry on room air was 88%, which improved with oxygen therapy to 95%. The patient was admitted to the hospital, where the infant received parenteral fluids and oxygen support. A chest x-ray revealed bilateral interstitial infiltrates and hyperaeration, with mild consolidation at the bases. Bronchodilator therapy was initiated with mixed results. A rapid viral antigen test yielded positive results for RSV (respiratory syncytial virus), confirming along with the clinical and x-ray findings that the patient had bronchiolitis. The patient remained in the hospital for 48 hours, and upon time of discharge had an improved respiratory rate with no signs of respiratory distress, was tolerating oral feeds, and had an oxygen saturation of 95% on room air.

Bronchiolitis is an inflammatory process of the smaller lower airways, usually caused by RSV. Bronchiolitis can progress to respiratory failure and potentially be fatal. RSV bronchiolitis is responsible for nearly 100,000 inpatient admissions, usually each winter and spring. Infants with congenital heart disease, chronic lung disease (usually former premature infants), and those with immunodeficiencies are usually at risk for more severe disease and poorer outcomes. Patients generally present with fever and upper respiratory tract infection, which is accompanied by tachypnea and wheezing. The diagnosis can be made clinically, but chest x-ray and viral antigen tests may aid in the diagnosis or in ruling out other causes. The goal of therapy is supportive care, usually achieved with oxygen and fluids; however, a significant number of patients require intensive care unit settings. Generally, the prognosis is excellent, but there may be an increased incidence of reactive airway disease subsequent to RSV infections.

QUESTIONS

45. Which of the following is a cause of bronchiolitis?
    A. RSV
    B. Adenovirus
    C. Influenzae
    D. Parainfluenzae
    E. All of the above

46. Which of the following is *not* traditionally used to treat bronchiolitis?
    A. Albuterol
    B. Amoxicillin
    C. Corticosteroids
    D. Ribavirin
    E. Oxygen

47. Apnea is a more frequent presentation of bronchiolitis among:
    A. Teenagers
    B. Infants
    C. Neonates
    D. School-age children

48. Which of the following may offer passive prophylaxis against RSV?
    A. Ribavirin
    B. Palivizumab (Synagis)
    C. DTaP
    D. Air purifiers

ID/CC: 2-year-old boy with persistent cough.

HPI: C.C., a 2-year-old Caucasian boy, presents with a nearly 6-month history of persistent cough. The cough occurs during the day and night and is "hacking," according to the mother. He was diagnosed with reactive airway disease 4 months ago and was given bronchodilators, which help him intermittently. His coughs seem to progressively worsen with each "cold" that he gets. The cough is forceful, and occasionally makes him vomit. He has had no prolonged fever, no ill contacts, and no recent travel. Mother is also concerned because he seems to be smaller than most children his age.

PMHx: Diagnosed with bronchiolitis at 12 months, repeated visits for upper respiratory infections over last few months. *Birth:* Born at home, SVD at term without complications.

PSHx: None   **Meds:** Albuterol PRN, over-the-counter cough medications

All: NKDA   **Immunizations:** UTD for age

DevHx: Reached milestones appropriately. *ROS:* no hemoptysis.

DietHx: History of formula intolerance ("formulas make his stools bulky and frothy")

SHx: Lives with parents and older brother, no smokers, no pets, attends daycare.

FHx: Maternal uncle died in adolescence from pneumonia.

VS: Temp 98.4°F, BP 90/50, HR 130, RR 36; Weight 10.2 kg (<3rd percentile)

PE: *Gen:* alert, cooperative, in no acute distress, passes a bulky/frothy stool while examining. *HEENT:* normal. *Chest:* scattered wheezes audible in all fields, localized coarse crackles in middle fields, slightly increased AP diameter of chest. *CV:* RR&R, normal S_1, S_2, no murmur, cap refill and pulses normal. *Abdomen:* mild distention, positive bowel sounds, no visceromegaly appreciated. *Skin:* no cyanosis, no edema.

THOUGHT QUESTIONS

- What is in your differential diagnosis?
- What elements of the history and physical would help in making a diagnosis?
- What diagnostic studies may help in making the diagnosis?

The differential diagnosis for chronic cough (defined as a persistent cough lasting greater than 3 weeks) can include the following: reactive airway disease, gastroesophageal reflux, foreign body aspiration, laryngotracheomalacia, congenital pulmonary anomalies, cystic fibrosis, ciliary dyskinesia syndromes, recurrent viral infections, atypical pneumonia/TB, and immunodeficiencies. Because of the wide range of diseases, history and physical examination can often narrow the diagnosis. History should characterize the cough via precipitating factors, patterns, and response to therapies. Associated symptoms and past medical problems should be ascertained. A review of systems, developmental, and environmental history should be obtained. The physical examination should be comprehensive. General appearance and developmental status should be noted. The exam should note any clubbing or evidence of nasal polyps, both which may suggest the pathologic cause. The chest exam should focus on the rate, ease of respiration, and adventitious sounds. Diagnostic studies should be driven by the history and physical exam, but may include pulse oximetry, PPD, CBC, sputum studies, chest and thoracic imaging, immune studies, and sweat chloride testing.

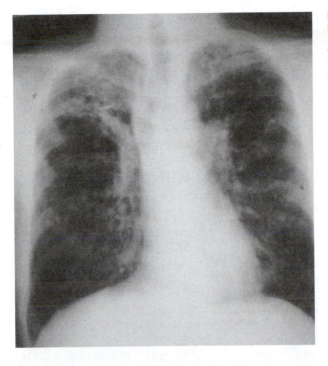

FIGURE 13 Marked chronic lung disease changes (fibrosis, bronchiectasis, and parenchymal loss) and characteristic "bleb" formation are seen in the adolescent boy with cystic fibrosis. Used with permission from Marino B, Snead K, McMillan J. Blueprints in Pediatrics, 2nd ed. Malden: Blackwell Science, Inc., 2001: 277.

CASE CONTINUED

A chest x-ray was performed, which revealed large airway infiltrates, patches of mild bronchiectasis, and marked hyperinflation. His history of feeding intolerance and bulky/frothy stools prompted a stool collection, which was markedly positive for fat. Further findings on physical exam revealed mild digital clubbing. A sweat chloride test result was 90 mEq/L (>60 is abnormal), and the diagnosis of cystic fibrosis was made. It was later learned that the maternal uncle had cystic fibrosis too.

Cystic fibrosis (CF) is a multisystem disease that results in disorders of the exocrine glands. Highly viscous secretions are the result of a defective chloride channel (CFTR: cystic fibrosis transmembrane receptor) and the subsequent insufficiency of water within the secretions. It is more prevalent in Caucasians, occurring in 1 in 2500 live births. The clinical manifestations are protean and include nasal polyps, pancreatic failure, and recurrent bronchopneumonia infections resulting from *Pseudomonas* species. Through multidisciplinary therapy and new advances, life expectancy has increased (median life span is approximately 30 years).

QUESTIONS

49. What is the inheritance pattern for CF?
    A. Autosomal dominant
    B. Autosomal recessive
    C. X-linked dominant
    D. X-linked recessive

50. Which of the following is least likely to be a complication of CF?
    A. Hemoptysis
    B. Pneumothorax
    C. Pancreatic cancer
    D. Male infertility
    E. Cirrhosis

51. Which of the following is usually pathognomonic for CF diagnosis in the neonate?
    A. Tachypnea
    B. Maculopapular rash
    C. Clubbing
    D. Meconium ileus
    E. None of the above

52. Which of the following are true regarding CF therapy/management?
    A. Pulmonary therapies are limited to DNAse mucolytics.
    B. Aminoglycosides are usually not indicated for bacterial infections.
    C. Pancreatic enzyme replacement may help achieve normal growth.
    D. Lung transplantation is not a viable option.

ID/CC: A 3-day-old male infant is brought in by his mother for "yellow skin."

HPI: According to his mother, P.J. has occasionally been a little "sleepy," but is otherwise acting well. There has been no fever, trouble breathing, or cyanosis. His mother's milk has just come in, and the baby seems to be feeding well. The yellow color appeared on his face on the day after birth, but has now deepened and progressed to the entire body as well as the eyes. Mother is worried that there is something wrong with her milk.

PMHx: *Birth:* Full term, normal spontaneous vaginal delivery (NSVD) at 39 2/7 wks. Mother is a 28-year-old Hispanic woman, G2, P2; prenatal labs all negative, an uncomplicated pregnancy with excellent prenatal care.

Meds: None   **All:** NKDA   **Immunizations:** Hepatitis B at birth

---

THOUGHT QUESTIONS

- What is your differential diagnosis?
- What further history or laboratory tests would you like to obtain for this jaundiced newborn?

Bilirubin, a pigment derived from the degradation of heme, must be conjugated in the liver into a form that can be excreted via the intestines. The newborn liver has impaired conjugation ability; therefore, most newborns develop a mild and temporary unconjugated (indirect) hyperbilirubinemia termed "physiologic jaundice." The differential diagnosis for prolonged or severe unconjugated hyperbilirubinemia includes factors that increase the accumulation of bilirubin, such as ABO or Rh hemolytic disease, polycythemia or extravascular blood collection, and factors that decrease its conjugation and excretion from the body, such as dehydration or intestinal obstruction. Conjugated (direct) hyperbilirubinemia is much less common, always pathologic, and most often caused by factors that impede the passage of bile through the liver.

A thorough history of the jaundiced infant's feeding and stooling habits, family history for hemolytic or hepatic disease, and a careful physical examination will help narrow the above differential. Laboratory tests, starting with a fractionated bilirubin level and blood type, should be performed judiciously, based on the suspected source of jaundice as suggested by history and physical exam.

CASE CONTINUED

Further history reveals that P.J. breastfeeds every 2 to 3 hours for 10 minutes per side. He has 4 to 5 wet diapers per day (normal: 6 to 8), and 3 to 4 stools (normal: 4 to 8), which are greenish and soft. There is no known family history of liver disease, hematologic disease, or genetic disorders. No one at home is ill.

VS: Temp 37.1°C (98.8°F), HR 150, RR 55; Weight 3.5 kg (70%); O_2 sat 99% on RA.

PE: *Gen:* icteric male newborn, sucking vigorously on mother's breast, who cries appropriately when examined. *HEENT:* icteric sclerae and mucus membranes, AFOSF, sutures normal, 4 × 6 cm soft resolving cephalohematoma on the left. Strong suck reflex. *Abdomen:* soft, nontender, normal active bowel sounds. The liver is palpable 1 cm below the costal margin, no spleen or other masses. *Neuro:* normal tone, intact Moro, grasp, suck. *Skin:* jaundiced to the ankles. Yellow color of skin is more easily visualized when you press on the skin to blanch it. Capillary refill is brisk. No petechiae, rashes, or bruising.

Labs: Mother's blood type: A+, baby's, blood type: O+. Direct Coombs' test negative, T bili 20.7, D bili 0.3, Hct 52 with normal morphology, normal reticulocyte count.

THOUGHT QUESTIONS

- What is your assessment of the most likely cause of jaundice in this newborn?
- How would you manage this infant?

Because there is no evidence to suggest hemolysis or serious illness on history or physical examination, this jaundiced newborn most likely has a form of physiologic jaundice exaggerated by factors such as mild dehydration from early breastfeeding and an extravascular blood collection (the cephalohematoma). In this case, the primary goal of therapy is to help the infant to eliminate excess bilirubin from the body until the period of physiologic jaundice has passed. Phototherapy is the standard treatment for moderate jaundice that approaches 20 mg/dL of total bilirubin. Ultraviolet light converts unconjugated bilirubin into several water-soluble stereoisomeric forms that can be excreted without conjugation. In addition, frequent feeds and adequate hydration are essential to ensure the efficient intestinal elimination of bilirubin from the body.

QUESTIONS

53. Treating hyperbilirubinemia with phototherapy is done primarily to prevent which of the following:
    A. Sepsis
    B. Hemolysis
    C. Permanent staining of the skin
    D. Kernicterus

54. All of the following characterize physiologic jaundice *except*:
    A. It begins before 24 hours of life.
    B. It peaks at 12–15 mg/dL.
    C. It is an unconjugated bilirubinemia.
    D. It resolves by the end of the first week of life.

55. Conjugated bilirubinemia, which is always pathologic, can be caused by all of the following *except*:
    A. Biliary atresia
    B. Breastfeeding
    C. Neonatal hepatitis
    D. Cystic fibrosis

56. To identify potentially significant ABO incompatibility, an infant's blood type and Coombs' reactivity is routinely determined if the mother is blood type:
    A. A+
    B. B+
    C. AB+
    D. O+

ID/CC: 15-minute-old newborn baby boy, born prematurely at 32 weeks' GA (gestational age), is brought to the intensive care nursery (ICN) with tachypnea.

HPI: R.D. is a 1430-gram baby boy born via caesarian section for maternal preeclampsia and breech presentation to a 31-year-old woman, G3, P2, blood type A+, serology (–), rubella immune, and hepatitis B surface antigen (–) who has had good prenatal care. The mother presented 2 days ago to the obstetric clinic complaining of a headache and was found to have an elevated blood pressure of 190/120. She was placed on appropriate antihypertensive medication but did not respond to the therapy. Her obstetricians thus decided to deliver the infant by C-section for maternal indications following a 48-hour course of betamethasone to enhance fetal lung maturity.

The infant was born blue, floppy, with poor tone and HR 60. The baby was resuscitated in the delivery room with 100% oxygen via face mask until pink with HR >100 and breathing spontaneously, and was then brought back to the ICN for further management. In the ICN, his face mask was briefly removed and he was noted to have a respiratory rate of 75 with moderate intercostal retractions, nasal flaring, and a blood saturation of 77% in room air (right arm).

THOUGHT QUESTIONS

- What is in this patient's differential diagnosis?
- Which test should be done to determine this baby's ability to ventilate the lungs?
- What additional blood tests should be ordered immediately?

The differential diagnosis in a premature newborn infant with respiratory distress should always include respiratory distress syndrome (RDS, or hyaline membrane disease), caused by a deficiency of surfactant in the alveoli. Additional causes in conjunction with RDS could include sepsis, pneumonia, pneumothorax, polycythemia, transient tachypnea of the newborn (from retained lung fluid), or any mass-occupying lesions or obstructions within the chest (e.g., congenital cystadenomatous malformations (CCAMs), pulmonary sequestration, lobar emphysema, congenital diaphragmatic hernia, vascular ring). The mass lesions are often identified during routine prenatal fetal ultrasound examination, but many go undiagnosed until birth.

Before birth, it is helpful to determine the amniotic fluid lecithin/sphingomyelin ratio (L:S ratio), which is a measure of lung maturity. A value greater than 2 generally indicates lungs with sufficient surfactant to sustain adequate lung volumes. After birth, an arterial blood gas (ABG) should be performed on this patient to measure the serum pCO_2, which assesses adequacy of ventilation. A blood gas obtained from a heelstick or vein is also acceptable, as pCO_2 values are fairly close to arterial values.

Additional blood tests should include a hematocrit, CBC with differential, and blood culture.

CASE CONTINUED

VS: Temp 97.5°F, BP 56/32 (MAP 40), HR 140, RR 75

PE: *Gen:* color pink, tachypneic infant with nasal flaring, moderate intercostal retractions, and occasional grunting. *HEENT:* fontanel soft/flat, no cleft palate. *Lungs:* minimal air movement bilaterally, slightly "crackly." *CV:* RR&R, normal S_1, S_2, no murmur, capillary refill time 2 sec. Remainder of exam normal for 32 weeks' GA.

Labs: ABG pH 7.20, pCO_2 70, pO_2 41, BE 0, Hct 51, CBC within normal limits, blood culture pending.

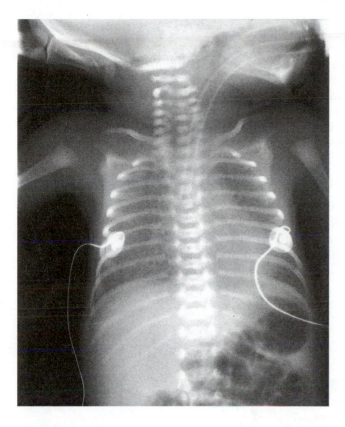

FIGURE 15 X-ray showing the features of respiratory distress syndrome. Used with permission from Rudolf M, Levene M. Paediatrics and Child Health. Oxford: Blackwell Science, Ltd., 1999: 248.

From the chest x-ray and ABG you determine that this premature infant has RDS and is not adequately ventilating his lungs (indicated by the primary respiratory acidosis with pCO_2 70 on ABG). The management of RDS involves exogenous replacement of artificial surfactant, maintenance of adequate functional residual capacity (FRC) using continuous positive airway pressure (CPAP) and/or intubation and mechanical ventilation. The comprehensive management of premature infants involves providing adequate nutrition, appropriate initiation of enteral feeds, maintenance of adequate blood volume, antibiotics to rule out sepsis, and monitoring for the risk of intracranial hemorrhage (ICH).

QUESTIONS

57. Which of the following chest x-ray findings is *not* associated with RDS?
    A. Low lung volumes
    B. Air bronchograms
    C. Pulmonary edema
    D. "Ground-glass" appearance of lung parenchyma

58. Which of the following cell types is responsible for the production of endogenous surfactant in the lung?
    A. Alveolar type I cells
    B. Alveolar type II cells
    C. Clara cells
    D. Ciliated tracheal cells

59. Which of the following is *not* a complication of exogenous surfactant therapy?
    A. Transient desaturation
    B. Hypoglycemia
    C. Pulmonary hemorrhage
    D. Pneumothorax

60. The benefits of antenatal maternal steroid administration when premature delivery is anticipated include which of the following?
    A. Decreased incidence of severe RDS
    B. Decreased incidence of intracranial hemorrhage
    C. Both A and B
    D. None of the above

ID/CC: 15-minute-old full-term newborn baby boy presents to the well-baby nursery with tachypnea.

HPI: P.D. is a 3430-gram baby boy born via caesarean section for failure to progress to a 31-year-old woman, G2, P2, blood type A+, serology (–), rubella immune, hepatitis B surface antigen (–), who has had good prenatal care. At delivery, the baby was blue but had a good cry and spontaneous respirations with Apgar scores of 9[1], 9[5] (2 for heart rate, 2 for respirations, 2 for reflexivity, 2 for tone, and 1 for color). The baby was warmed and dried and taken to the well-baby nursery for recovery. At 15-minutes' age he was still noted to be cyanotic and had blood oxygen saturation values of 80% (right arm) and 100% (right leg), and an ABG (right arm) pH 7.44, pCO_2 35, pO_2 35, BE 0, in room air.

VS: Temp 97.9°F, BP 65/40 (MAP 50), HR 150, RR 100

PE: *Gen:* awake, looking around, cyanotic, especially head and shoulders as compared to lower extremities. *Lungs:* good aeration bilaterally, no rales, rhonchi, or wheezing. *CV:* RR&R, prominent precordial heave, single loud S_2. No murmur. *Abdomen:* soft, nondistended, positive bowel sounds, no hepatomegaly or splenomegaly. *Ext:* equal peripheral pulses in brachial, femoral, and dorsalis pedis arteries.

THOUGHT QUESTIONS

- What is in this patient's differential diagnosis?
- What simple (nonradiologic) test can be performed to differentiate between pulmonary versus congenital heart disease?
- What is the significance of the cyanosis of the upper extremity and the differential in preductal and postductal saturations?

The differential diagnosis in a term newborn with tachypnea includes transient tachypnea of the newborn (TTN, retained lung fluid), sepsis, pneumonia, pneumothorax, chest masses or obstructions (e.g., CCAMs, pulmonary sequestration, lobar emphysema, congenital diaphragmatic hernia, vascular rings), persistent pulmonary hypertension (PPHN), and congenital heart disease. In this infant with cyanosis and a preductal and postductal saturation difference, PPHN and congenital heart disease should be considered. The congenital heart lesions that present as a cyanotic infant with tachypnea are those that lead to pulmonary overcirculation such as transposition of the great arteries (TGA), truncus arteriosus, and total anomalous pulmonary venous return (TAPVR).

The simple test to help differentiate a pulmonary versus congenital heart defect is a hyperoxia challenge. In this maneuver, the baby is placed in a 100% oxygen hood and an arterial blood gas is drawn. With pulmonary disease, the PaO_2 can be expected to rise >150 torr, whereas in congenital heart defects it should remain <50 torr.

The significance of upper extremity cyanosis and higher postductal compared to preductal saturations suggests that oxygenated blood from the pulmonary circulation is entering the descending aorta through a patent ductus arteriosus.

CASE CONTINUED

You perform a hyperoxia challenge test revealing a PaO$_2$ of 39 in 100% oxygen hood and determine that this infant must have transposition of the great arteries.

> ### THOUGHT QUESTIONS
> - What is the next important radiological test to perform?
> - What is the importance of the ductus arteriosus in TGA?

An echocardiogram is important to confirm the diagnosis of TGA and to ascertain whether an associated ventricular septal defect also exists. In cases of severe hypoxia in which the ventricular septum is intact, it may be necessary to perform an emergency atrial balloon septostomy (Rashkind procedure) to improve atrial mixing.

TGA is a ductal-dependent lesion, which means that patency of the ductus arteriosus is critical to survival. In these cases, it is important to start an infusion of prostaglandin PGE$_1$ to maintain ductal patency until complete surgical repair with an arterial switch can be performed.

CASE CONTINUED

The baby was started on PGE$_1$ and a surgical arterial switch was done to correct the defect. The baby had an uncomplicated course and was discharged to home 3 weeks later on full feeds.

QUESTIONS

61. The classic chest x-ray finding associated with TGA is:
    - A. "Boot-shaped" heart
    - B. "Snowman" appearance of heart
    - C. "Egg on a string" appearance of heart
    - D. "Sail" sign

62. The electrocardiogram (ECG) in TGA has an electrical force axis which is:
    - A. Left axis deviation with left ventricular hypertrophy
    - B. Right axis deviation with right ventricular hypertrophy
    - C. Superior axis deviation
    - D. Between 180° and 270°

63. Tetralogy of Fallot consists of all of the following *except*:
    - A. Pulmonary stenosis
    - B. Right ventricular hypertrophy
    - C. Atrial septal defect
    - D. Overriding aorta
    - E. Ventricular septal defect

64. The clinical finding of low blood pressures in the lower compared to upper extremities suggests which of the following congenital heart lesions?
    - A. Tricuspid atresia
    - B. Pulmonary atresia
    - C. Coarctation of the aorta
    - D. Tetralogy of Fallot

ID/CC: 4-week-old baby boy presents to urgent care clinic with vomiting for past 2 days.

HPI: M.V. was born slightly prematurely at 35 weeks' GA by caesarean section for severe variable decelerations to a 32-year-old woman, G1, P1, A+, serology (–), rubella immune, hepatitis B (–), VDRL (–), who had good prenatal care. She had a routine 20-week prenatal sonogram that revealed a normal fetus and amniotic fluid. At delivery, baby M.V. was found to have a nuchal cord × 2 but was born vigorous, with Apgar scores of 6 and 9 following brief blow-by O_2 and a birth weight of 2280 grams. He was discharged to home after good breastfeeding was established in 2 days. He had a normal 2-week visit, at which time his weight was noted to be 2290 gram with a normal physical examination. His mother states that for the past 2 days he has been vomiting up most of his formula about 30 minutes after his feeding, and over the past day has had very forceful green vomits. He has been breastfed every 3 to 4 hours and his mother feels he has a good suck and swallow. He had a normal stooling pattern with four stools per day of mustard yellow and seedy consistency, although this morning his mother noted a single dark-brown colored stool. He now feeds for only about 5 minutes per breast and vomits most of the quantity, which has turned green, within 10 minutes. Today his weight is 2680 gram.

THOUGHT QUESTIONS

- What is the significance of the green vomitus?
- What is in this patient's differential diagnosis?

The significance of the green vomitus indicates that it is bilious in nature. Bilious vomiting indicates an obstructed bowel distal to the ampulla of Vater, the point where bile empties into the duodenum.

The differential diagnosis of a newborn infant with vomiting can be divided into two categories: bilious and nonbilious. Bilious vomiting generally involves conditions with partial or complete bowel obstruction such as malrotation, volvulus, Ladd's bands, Hirschsprung disease, incarcerated hernia, torsion of Meckel's diverticulum, and intestinal atresia. Nonbilious vomiting in a newborn is largely due to gastroesophageal reflux, cow or soy milk protein intolerance, and pyloric stenosis. Although rare, nonbilious vomiting may also occur in esophageal atresia, but is usually diagnosed immediately after initiation of feeds.

PMHx:/PSHx: None **Meds:** None **All:** NKDA

FHx: No family history of gastrointestinal disorders.

SHx: Lives at home with mother and father. At home with mother during the day.

VS: Temp 98.5°F, BP 57/24 (MAP 30), HR 79, RR 28

PE: *Gen:* awake, alert, and crying. *HEENT:* mucous membranes moist, throat nonerythematous. *Lungs:* clear bilaterally. *Abdomen:* soft, moderately distended, minimal bowel sounds, cries during exam, especially with palpation of abdomen; no masses or hepatosplenomegaly. *Rectum:* anus patent, no fissures noted. Stool test guaiac negative. *Skin:* slight pallor, capillary refill time 5 to 6 sec.

THOUGHT QUESTIONS

- What aspect of the physical examination is particularly concerning?
- What radiological test would be helpful at this time?

The compromised hemodynamic state (low blood pressure, prolonged capillary refill time of 5 to 6 seconds) is of concern because it suggests an infant who is in shock. Of primary importance will be to resuscitate the infant and to establish adequate perfusion concurrent with determining the cause of the clinical symptoms.

An initial KUB x-ray is a reasonable initial study to obtain, but when a possible obstructive cause is suspected, an upper GI series with a small bowel follow through should be performed. If a malrotation/volvulus is suspected, an abdominal ultrasound may also help confirm the diagnosis.

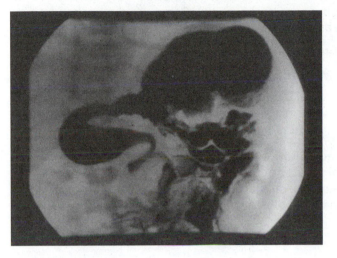

FIGURE 17 Malrotation with volvulus on upper GI series with small bowel follow through. Note the contrast in small bowel is limited entirely to the left of midline, indicating malrotation. Also note corkscrew appearance of contrast, indicating volvulus within proximal small bowel.

CASE CONTINUED

Labs: X-rays: *KUB:* gas in the stomach with paucity of air in the intestine. No free-air noted. *Upper GI series:* contrast within stomach and extending only to level of the ligament of Treitz, located in the right upper quadrant. *Abdominal US:* cecum located in the left lower quadrant.

You determine this baby has a malrotation with an associated volvulus.

QUESTIONS

65. The diagnosis of malrotation is definitive because:
    A. The ligament of Treitz is abnormally located in the right quadrant.
    B. The cecum is abnormally located in the left quadrant.
    C. There is a history of bilious vomiting.
    D. Only A and B.
    E. All of the above.

66. The next step after confirming the diagnosis of malrotation with volvulus is to:
    A. Consult pediatric gastroenterologists to request an emergent endoscopic procedure.
    B. Consult pediatric surgeons for emergent surgical intervention.
    C. Place an orogastric tube for decompression of the bowels and repeat an upper GI series in 4 to 6 hours.
    D. Perform a barium enema to note the abnormal placement of the cecum in the left lower quadrant.

67. Malrotation with associated volvulus often results in bowel ischemia or infarction due to twisting of the mesenteric blood supply, which includes the:
    A. Superior gastric artery
    B. Inferior gastric artery
    C. Superior mesenteric artery
    D. Inferior mesenteric artery

68. The primary metabolic derangement often associated with malrotation and volvulus is:
    A. Respiratory acidosis
    B. Respiratory alkalosis
    C. Metabolic acidosis
    D. Metabolic alkalosis

ID/CC: 6-week-old infant brought to emergency room at midnight by parents who complain he is "breathing fast and very sleepy."

HPI: Parents report that S.T. was well until about 2 days ago when he started becoming increasingly "fussy" and showed decreased interest in feeding. Tonight, he has also become tachypneic but is less fussy. In fact, he seems to be sleeping more than usual and is not feeding at all. He has had no fevers or other signs of illness (no runny nose, coughing, vomiting, diarrhea, or rashes) and has not been exposed to anyone who was recently ill. There has also been no history of trauma or falls.

PMHx: *Birth:* unremarkable with normal pregnancy and spontaneous vaginal delivery (SVD) at 39 weeks' GA and Apgar scores of 9 and 9 (at 1 and 5 minutes, respectively). Baby was discharged home on day of life 3 and had a normal 2-week checkup as outpatient.

Meds: None **All:** NKDA **FHx:** No history of metabolic or endocrine disorders in the family.

SHx: Lives at home with mother, father, no pets. Mother at home daily (not working).

VS: Temp 98.8°F, BP 65/45, HR 280, RR 70; 98% O_2 saturation on room air; Weight 4405 gram (birth weight 3810 gram).

PE: *Gen:* sleeping quietly, tachypneic, slightly ashen color. *HEENT:* normocephalic; anterior fontanelle soft/flat; otherwise normal. *Lungs:* clear to auscultation bilaterally; sternal and intercostal retractions. *CV:* tachycardia, regular rhythm; normal S_1, S_2, no murmurs. *Abdomen:* soft, no distention, positive bowel sounds, liver edge palpable 4 cm below costal margin; no splenomegaly; no masses. *Ext:* pulses full in upper and lower extremities. Remainder of exam normal.

THOUGHT QUESTIONS

- What is in this patient's differential diagnosis?
- What is the significance of this heart rate in an infant at rest?
- What is the most appropriate *non*hematologic test to perform?

Tachycardia often accompanies pain or agitation in an infant (sinus tachycardia), but in an infant who is resting comfortably you must consider a pathologic cause. Fever can also cause increased heart rate, but usually to a lower extent (low 200s). Sepsis should always be a strong consideration in an infant this age with poor feeding and abnormal vital signs. Other possibilities to consider include dehydration, anemia, hypovolemia (i.e., blood loss), or toxic ingestion (accidental or through breast milk). However, these factors rarely cause an increase in heart rate much above 200.

The extremely high level of tachycardia in this patient suggests that he could have a tachyarrhythmia, such as any type of supraventricular tachycardia (SVT). Whenever an abnormal heart rate is detected in an infant, special attention should be paid to assessing the patient's hemodynamic stability before proceeding with the diagnostic workup. This includes examination of pulses, skin color and perfusion, and oxygenation. Because this patient appears well compensated in these areas, you may proceed with the further investigation into the cause for his tachycardia.

This infant should have laboratory tests to evaluate for sepsis because of his young age and ill appearance. In addition, because of the suspicion of arrhythmia, the most useful supplemental diagnostic test to perform at this time would be an electrocardiogram (ECG) looking for presence or absence of P waves and any signs of reentrant phenomena.

CASE CONTINUED

Labs: CBC: WBC 15,000, no bands, 40% segs, 40% lymphs; platelets 320,000, hct. 41 g/dL. Blood culture sent. ABG (right arm): 7.22/33/95/–6 in room air chest x-ray: normal lung fields and heart size. ECG: see Fig 18.

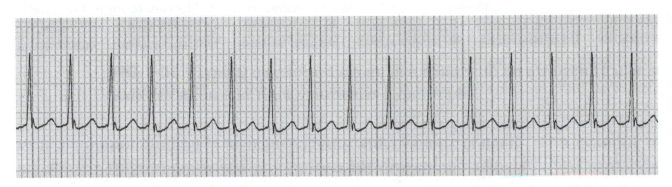

FIGURE 18 Supraventricular tachycardia. Normal QRS complex tachycardia at a rate of over 200 beats per minute. Note lack of visible P waves.

Based on the reassuring sepsis workup and the ECG results, you determine this patient has SVT, the most common type of arrhythmia in children. The base deficit of –6 on the ABG probably reflects some compromise to proper perfusion to the systemic circulation and thus warrants immediate correction of the underlying arrhythmia.

QUESTIONS

69. A quick review of the classification of this atrial tachyarrhythmia yields two types of SVT: automatic and reentrant. The most common reentry SVT is:
    A. Atrioventricular reentry tachycardia—Wolff-Parkinson-White (WPW) syndrome
    B. Atrioventricular nodal reentry tachycardia
    C. Atrial flutter
    D. Atrial fibrillation
    E. Sinoatrial nodal reentry tachycardia

70. Which of the following is *true*?
    A. P waves are always absent in SVT.
    B. A delta wave on ECG represents an initial slurred ventricular conduction delay and is called preexcitation.
    C. SVT only occurs in infants.
    D. SVT is associated with prolonged PR interval.

71. All of the following may be used to treat SVT in infants *except*:
    A. Ice bag to face
    B. Adenosine
    C. Digoxin
    D. Verapamil
    E. Synchronized DC cardioversion

72. In patients with conduction disorders due to bypass tracts (e.g., WPW syndrome), antegrade conduction occurs through which of the following?
    A. Sinoatrial node
    B. Atrioventricular node
    C. His bundle
    D. Kent bundle

ID/CC: Full-term newborn baby presents with ambiguous genitalia.

HPI: A.H. is a 3250-gram baby born via SVD through clear amniotic fluid to a 22-year-old woman, G1, P0, A+, antibody (–), rubella immune, hepatitis B surface antigen (–), VDRL nonreactive, group B *Streptococcus* (–), who had good prenatal care. At birth the infant was pink, vigorous, with sponta-neous respirations and a loud cry, and had Apgar scores of 9 and 9 at 1 and 5 minutes, respectively. After warming and drying the infant, a pediatrician was consulted to the delivery room to examine the baby's genitalia. The parents were reassured that the baby was in stable condition, but that a more thorough examination was necessary to determine the exact gender.

PMHx:/PSHx: None   **Meds:** None   **All:** NKDA

FHx: No history of ambiguous genitalia or other endocrine disorders in the family.

SHx: Mother and father live together.

VS: Temp 97°F, BP 65/44, HR 120, RR 40

PE: *Gen:* awake, alert, pink. *HEENT:* normocephalic, ant. fontanel soft/flat. Eyes PERRLA, normal fundi, normal ears. *Lungs:* clear bilaterally. *CV:* RR&R, normal S_1, S_2, no murmur. *Abdomen:* soft, nondistended, positive bowel sounds, no masses. Normal liver edge. Kidneys of normal size palpable bilaterally. *GU:* small 1.5 cm soft tissue resembling penile tissue superior to bifid scrotum versus fused labia. *Skin:* no discolored spots or patches.

Labs: Na 122, K 3.5, Cl 100, CO_2 25, BUN 10, Cr 0.5

THOUGHT QUESTIONS

- What is in this patient's differential diagnosis?
- What is a key maneuver to perform on physical examination to help determine the cause of ambiguous genitalia?

The differential diagnosis of ambiguous genitalia is first divided into two major categories: virilized female, or inadequate virilization of a male. The causes of virilized female include congenital adrenal hyperplasia (CAH), androgenic drug exposure (e.g., progestins), true hermaphroditism (XO/XY karyotype), or maternal virilizing adrenal tumor. The causes of inadequate virilization of a male include steroid and steroid precursor deficiency, dysgenetic testes, Leydig cell hypoplasia, testicular feminization, partial androgen insensitivity, and 5α-reductase deficiency.

The key maneuver to focus upon during physical examination is to attempt to palpate gonads. Palpable gonads are nearly always testes and indicate that incomplete development of a male has occurred. Similarly, an ultrasound may be helpful to detect whether a uterus, cervix, and vagina are present.

CASE CONTINUED

Repeat examination reveals no palpable gonads and abdominal ultrasound reveals the presence of a uterus and ovaries.

You determine that this patient must be a virilized female and obtain a genetics and urologic surgery consult to aid the family in deciding whether to rear the infant as a boy or a girl. You are aware that this decision is largely based on the prognosis of the underlying hormonal defect and the feasibility of genital reconstruction; today most patients are able to be hormonally replaced, have surgery, and be raised as girls.

QUESTIONS

73. The most common cause of CAH is a deficiency of which of the following?
    A. 17-hydroxylase
    B. 21-hydroxylase
    C. 11-hydroxylase
    D. 17-hydroxyprogesterone

74. The diagnosis of CAH is made by measuring an elevation in which of the following?
    A. 17-hydroxylase
    B. 21-hydroxylase
    C. 11-hydroxylase
    D. 17-hydroxyprogesterone

75. A key difference between 21-hydroxylase deficiency and 11-hydroxylase deficiency is that, unlike 21-hydroxylase deficiency, 11-hydroxylase deficiency is associated with:
    A. Hypernatremia
    B. Hypotension
    C. Cortisol overproduction
    D. No ambiguity of genitalia

76. The treatment of 21-hydroxylase deficiency includes administration of all the following *except*:
    A. Mineralocorticoid therapy
    B. Cortisol therapy
    C. Surgical treatment
    D. Testosterone

ID/CC: 10-year-old boy with a 2-day history of fever and abdominal pain.

HPI: A.A. has been experiencing abdominal pain for 2 days. His pain, "in the lower part of my belly, and near my belly-button," is worse when he tries to sit up, and he prefers to lie still in bed. He was given acetaminophen without any resolution. He has been vomiting since last night (no blood or bile) and had initial diarrhea on the first day of his illness. This morning his parents noticed that he had a fever (measured in the axilla at 101.8°F), but that his pain is relatively improved.

PMHx: Asthma (hospitalized once for exacerbation); otherwise, within normal limits.

Meds: Acetaminophen as above, herbal tea   **All:** NKDA

THOUGHT QUESTIONS
- What further questions would you ask as part of history?
- What is your differential diagnosis at this point?

Abdominal pain is a very common complaint in the pediatric population. When assessing a patient, it is important to ask questions regarding the specifics of the symptom (the quality and temporal characteristics of the pain, the exacerbating and relieving factors). Other important aspects of the history include a thorough diet history, travel history, history of trauma/ingestions, stooling habits, family history, sexual behavior history, a thorough review of symptoms, and behavioral/environmental history (including ill contacts).

A particularly thorough history should be obtained because the differential diagnosis for abdominal pain is extensive. In pediatrics, common causes for acute abdominal pain account for nearly 90% of diagnoses. These include viral gastroenteritis, bacterial enterocolitis, food poisoning, dietary indiscretion, appendicitis, UTI, and group A streptococcal pharyngitis. More uncommon causes include pelvic inflammatory disease (PID), lower lobe pneumonia, insulin-dependent diabetes mellitus (IDDM), obstructive disease, intussusception, perforated bowel, trauma, and conversion reactions.

CASE CONTINUED

Further history reveals anorexia and no bowel movements over the last 24 hours, no ill contacts or new food sources, and a negative review of symptoms.

VS: Temp 101°F, BP 130/65, HR 100, RR 30

PE: *Gen:* supine on table, appears uncomfortable but in no acute distress. *HEENT:* dry oral mucosa, otherwise noncontributory. *Lungs:* clear to auscultation, no crackles. *CV:* RR&R mild tachycardia, normal S_1, S_2, no murmur, otherwise normal pulses, CRT <2 sec. *Abdomen:* nondistended, hypoactive bowel sounds in all areas, mild guarding, pain on superficial palpation in periumbilical area, tympanic abdomen, no masses. *GU:* Tanner stage 1 to 2, normal external male genitalia, no swelling or masses.

THOUGHT QUESTIONS

- Are there any other components of the physical examination that you would like to perform?
- What laboratory tests or imaging studies, if any, would you obtain?

CASE CONTINUED

A urinalysis is performed that reveals no organisms, few WBCs and few RBCs. Based on his improving abdominal pain and clinical picture, the patient is diagnosed with an acute gastroenteritis of a likely viral origin, receives parenteral rehydration, acetaminophen for his pain and fever, and instructions on when to return to the office. He returns late that evening with persistent fever, anorexia, and worse abdominal pain. His examination now reveals pain localizing to his right lower quadrant, which increases when he is asked to move in bed. His WBC count is 19,000 with a left shift, and an abdominal computed tomography (CT) scan reveals a perforated appendix with evidence of diffuse peritonitis.

Appendicitis is generally a clinical diagnosis; however, laboratory values and imaging may augment clinical suspicion. In the case above, a thorough physical for the patient with acute abdominal pain should include a rectal exam to detect tenderness or a mass. Laboratory examination may reveal a moderately increased WBC count with left shift and mild pyuria or hematuria on urinalysis. Abdominal ultrasound can be used to identify an inflamed appendix; however, focused appendiceal CT scanning recently has been shown to be highly specific and sensitive in children with appendicitis.

QUESTIONS

77. The typical pediatric patient with appendicitis can present with which of the following?
   A. Fever, emesis, anorexia
   B. Periumbilical pain
   C. Right lower quadrant pain, guarding
   D. Obturator and psoas signs
   E. All of the above

78. Conditions that may mimic appendicitis include
   A. Lower lobe pneumonia
   B. *Yersinia* enterocolitis
   C. Urinary tract infection
   D. Diabetic ketoacidosis
   E. All of the above

79. Which of the following statements is *true*?
   A. The appendix typically perforates 12 to 24 hours after pain begins.
   B. The incidence of perforation in young children and toddlers is low.
   C. The retrocecal appendix usually induces pain well before perforation occurs.
   D. Wound infections, abscesses, and longer hospitalizations are associated with perforation.

80. Which of the following statements is *true*?
   A. Atypical presentation of appendicitis is quite rare in childhood.
   B. Diagnosis of appendicitis is established primarily by imaging.
   C. Rectal exam is rarely helpful in establishing the diagnosis of appendicitis.
   D. Appendicitis is the most common indication for abdominal surgery in childhood.
   E. Commonly, the majority of children with appendicitis are less than 5 years old.

ID/CC: 6-year-old boy with vomiting and worsening abdominal pain.

HPI: M.D. presents with 2 days of vomiting and worsening abdominal pain. His vomiting is non-bloody, nonbilious, and the pain is epigastric and "near his belly button." The pain is not relieved by position or vomiting. He has no fever, cough, rhinorrhea, or diarrhea. His mother states that he has been unable to tolerate any oral intake since yesterday, but he is still urinating regularly. Some of the children at his school are ill. This morning he seems to be quite uncomfortable and very tired.

PMHx: No prior hospitalization, evaluated several times for acute gastroenteritis.

Meds: None **All:** NKDA

SHx: Attends kindergarten, lives with parents, no smokers, no pets.

DietHx: "Usually eats like a horse, but never gains any weight!"

VS: Temp 99.8°F, BP 80/45, HR 140, RR 40

PE: *Gen:* lethargic, thin boy, breathing with difficulty, looks ill. *HEENT:* NCAT, extraocular movement intact (EOMI), PERRL, mucous membranes are dry. *Neck:* supple. *Lungs:* tachypneic and labored breathing, no crackles or wheeze appreciated. *CV:* tachycardic, RR&R, normal S_1, S_2, no murmur, capillary refill time 3.5 sec. *Abdomen:* decreased bowel sounds, periumbilical and epigastric tenderness; guarding. No visceromegaly appreciated. *Skin:* dry, no cyanosis, clubbing, or edema; decreased turgor.

THOUGHT QUESTIONS

- What further components of the history or physical examination would you like to explore?
- What signs and symptoms of dehydration are present in this patient?
- What is in your differential diagnosis at this point?
- What are some immediate measures to take in this patient?

When faced with the patient with acute abdominal pain and vomiting, obtaining a thorough history should include eliciting specifics regarding the pain, emesis, stool habits, and dietary habits/appetite. Prior surgery, a family history, travel history, and a review of symptoms will aid in the diagnosis. The physical examination findings in this patient that indicate dehydration include the vital signs—tachycardia, tachypnea, weight loss, hypotension (in decompensated/severe cases)—and poor skin turgor, dry mucous membranes, lethargy, and prolonged capillary refill time.

This patient appears to be quite ill and facing decompensated shock. The differential diagnosis includes septic shock/meningitis, severe acute gastroenteritis, metabolic or endocrine disorders (diabetic ketoacidosis, adrenal insufficiency), toxic ingestion, GI disorders (appendicitis, perforation, pancreatitis), and trauma. Immediate measures would include assessment of the ABCs including airway/breathing support and volume resuscitation (20 mL/kg of normal saline or lactated Ringer's solution), and appropriate monitoring of vital signs. Laboratory studies may include a CBC, blood gas measurement, serum electrolytes and glucose levels, urinalysis, and blood/urine for culture. Administration of empiric antibiotics should not be delayed in suspected cases of septic shock.

CASE CONTINUED

Upon assessing the ABCs, this noticeably ill appearing child was given aggressive fluids for his apparent dehydration. An astute nurse noticed a fruity odor to his breath. His electrolyte panel yielded: sodium of 155, chloride of 119, bicarbonate of 5, with an anion gap of 31, and a glucose of 495. Arterial blood gas revealed a pH of 7.12, and PCO_2 of 18. His urine was positive for glucose and ketones. Based upon his clinical presentation, the patient was transferred to the intensive care unit for further management of diabetic ketoacidosis. Further questioning yielded a positive family history for type 1 diabetes mellitus, and a review of symptoms revealed symptoms of polyuria, polydipsia, and polyphagia over the last several months.

Diabetes mellitus is the most common life-threatening pediatric endocrine disorder. Diabetic ketoacidosis (DKA) occurs with severe insulin deficiency, when excess ketone production (due to a lack of glucose utilization) overwhelms the blood's native buffering capacity. The result is a profound hyperglycemia, dehydration, metabolic acidosis, and lethargy. The mainstays of treatment of DKA include restoration of fluid volume, inhibition of lipolysis/return to glucose utilization, replacement of body salts, and correction of acidosis. The management of diabetes and its complications requires a multidisciplinary approach involving medical, nutritional, behavioral, and environmental interventions.

QUESTIONS

81. DKA presents with which of the following acid-base abnormalities?
    A. Metabolic alkalosis w/compensatory respiratory acidosis
    B. Metabolic acidosis w/compensatory respiratory alkalosis
    C. Respiratory acidosis w/compensatory metabolic alkalosis
    D. Respiratory alkalosis w/compensatory metabolic acidosis

82. Which of the following statements about DKA is *false*?
    A. Symptoms of hypoglycemia are due to catecholamine release.
    B. Hypokalemia is often the result of decreased serum pH level.
    C. Ketonuria will be present until the catabolic state is reversed.
    D. It can be triggered by inadequate insulin dosing.
    E. All of the above.

83. All of the following are true regarding type I diabetes mellitus *except*:
    A. Becomes clinically significant after 25% of B-cell function destroyed
    B. Anti-islet cell antibodies may be present
    C. May be complicated (long-term) by small and large vessel disease
    D. May be managed via insulin, diet/exercise therapy, and blood sugar monitoring
    E. May be associated with HLA DR3 and -DR4 antigens

84. Which of the following is true of type II diabetes mellitus?
    A. It is caused by excessive corticosteroid synthesis.
    B. Patients may commonly be thin and underweight.
    C. Patients very rarely present with skin findings.
    D. It is characterized by insulin resistance.
    E. It must be managed with insulin therapy.

ID/CC: 16-year-old boy with scrotal swelling and pain.

HPI: T.T. presents this evening to the emergency department with several hours of worsening pain and swelling of his scrotal area. The pain began late this afternoon and is worsened by any movement. He also complains of nausea and has vomited twice in the waiting room. He has had no fever, no dysuria, and no urinary urgency. He confides that he has become sexually active, and is afraid that this is a result of recent unprotected intercourse.

PMHx: Exercise-induced asthma **PSHx:** None **Meds:** Albuterol inhaler as needed

All: Penicillin **FHx:** Noncontributory

SHx: Lives at home with parents and older sister, 10th grade honor student, plays soccer, denies any toxic habits or exposures.

VS: Temp 98.8°F, BP 135/75, HR 120, RR 32

PE: *Gen:* anxious, lying on table. *HEENT:* within normal limits. *Chest:* slightly tachypneic, clear to auscultation. *CV:* tachycardic, RR&R normal S_1, S_2, no murmur. *Abdomen:* bowel sounds, mild suprapubic tenderness; otherwise, soft, nondistended/nontender, no masses. *Ext/Back:* no flank or side pain. *Skin:* no rashes, skin warm with no rash. *GU:* Tanner stage 5 external genitalia, swelling and redness of the right hemiscrotum, pain upon movement or palpation of the entire right testis, absent right cremasteric reflex, no relief of pain upon elevation of the scrotum. *ROS:* no weight loss, no recurrent fever, no rash, no discharge.

THOUGHT QUESTIONS

- What is your differential diagnosis at this point?
- What components of the history and physical examination help narrow this diagnosis?
- What diagnostic studies may help in the diagnosis?

For the patient who presents with scrotal swelling and pain, the differential diagnosis should include traumatic injury, torsion of the testis or appendix testis, incarcerated hernia, hydrocele, epididymitis, scrotal abscess, Henoch-Schönlein purpura, and leukemic infiltrate of the testis. Questions regarding pain (quality, location, timing/onset, radiation, and alleviating or precipitating factors) and a thorough review of systems can help narrow the diagnosis. In any adolescent, "HEADS" questions should be asked, regarding **H**ome life and family relationships, **E**ducation and school/vocation interests, **A**ctivities, **D**iet and nutrition, **D**epression and emotional health, **S**exuality and sexual activity, **S**ubstance use/abuse, and **S**afety and self-care. On physical examination, localization of the pain near the upper pole of the testis with a tender nodule may suggest torsion of the appendix testis, the most common cause of acute scrotal swelling and pain in the preadolescent male. Absent cremasteric reflex, associated with an exquisitely tender and slightly retracted testis, indicates a testicular torsion and is a surgical emergency. Epididymitis is associated with scrotal pain (which radiates along the spermatic cord into the flank and is relieved by lifting the scrotum), fever, and symptoms of frequency/urgency and dysuria.

In many patients, a definitive diagnosis cannot be discerned from history and physical examination, so imaging may be necessary to depict anatomy and blood flow. High-resolution color Doppler ultrasonography can greatly aid diagnosis, and is the procedure of choice in examining the acutely painful scrotum with unclear cause.

CASE CONTINUED

Based on the patient's history and positive physical findings, he was clinically diagnosed with testicular torsion. The patient was promptly referred for surgical management, and the right testis was salvaged. At his 2-week postoperative visit and in an appropriately confidential manner, you counsel him regarding safe sex practices, sexually transmitted diseases (STDs) and pregnancy.

QUESTIONS

85. Testicular torsion:
    A. occurs most commonly in preadolescent males (ages 9 to 12).
    B. can be associated with the "blue-dot" sign.
    C. can be treated with analgesics and observation.
    D. may result from an absent or narrow posterior mesenteric attachment.

86. Which of the following may cause painless scrotal swelling?
    A. Varicocele
    B. Hydrocele
    C. Testicular tumor
    D. Inguinal hernia
    E. All of the above

87. A 15-year-old boy presents with slight testicular pain and swelling of his scrotum over 3 days. He has had fever and last week suffered from parotid gland swelling. What is his likely diagnosis?
    A. Trauma
    B. Torsion of the appendix testis
    C. Mumps orchitis
    D. Idiopathic scrotal edema

88. Which of the following regarding cryptorchidism is true?
    A. It is less common in premature males than term males.
    B. There is no risk for malignancy.
    C. By age 1 year, most cases will have resolved.
    D. Hormone therapy is more successful than surgery.

ID/CC: 7-month-old with indigestion.

HPI: E.S. is a 7-month-old boy having "cramps" for the past several weeks. His parents state that they think that he is experiencing pain from indigestion, as he has been "repeatedly drawing his arms and legs up to his belly" and subsequently crying during these episodes. He has been feeding well, without fever, vomiting, or diarrhea. The "cramps" seem to occur in clusters, particularly when he is about to fall asleep and occasionally after a meal. The parents feel that this may be a result of introducing solid foods to him last month. They have tried simethicone drops without any resolution.

PMHx: NSVD at term without complications. **Meds:** Simethicone drops

All: NKDA **Immunizations:** UTD **FHx:** Noncontributory

DevHx: Maintains head supported, unable to sit independently, not yet babbling, not yet transferring objects. *ROS:* Noncontributory.

DietHx: Age-appropriate solids introduced at 5 months, breastfeeding.

VS: Temp 98.8°F, BP 90/50, HR 110, RR 26

PE: *Gen:* supine on table, alert/will regard face, and in no apparent distress. *HEENT:* nondysmorphic, NCAT, EOMI, PERRL, tympanic membranes within normal limits. *Lungs:* normal exam with no crackles or wheeze. *CV:* normal exam with no murmur, pulses and capillary refill time normal. *Abdomen:* bowel sounds; soft, no distention/no tenderness, no visceromegaly. *Neuro:* normal tone and reflexes, grossly nonfocal exam.

THOUGHT QUESTIONS

- What developmental milestones have not been appropriately met by this patient?
- What is in your differential diagnosis at this point?
- What further components of the physical examination or history would you explore?

The 7-month-old infant should be able to sit independently with adequate head and trunk support, to transfer grasped objects from one hand to the other, and begin some monosyllabic babbling. The differential diagnosis for this patient may include colic, constipation, gastroesophageal reflux, or other episodic events such as breath-holding spells or benign myoclonic activity. The associated developmental delay in this child, however, may also suggest an underlying neurologic problem manifesting as seizures. Further questions to ask may be related to the nature of the episodes: association with fever or feeds, relieving or exacerbating factors, relation to eating or sleeping, associated symptoms (vomiting, pallor, cyanosis, posturing), status of the child after the episode (alert, drowsy, altered consciousness). Aspects of the thorough physical examination include proper evaluation of the growth parameters, examining the skin for any lesions suggestive of neurocutaneous disorders, and eye grounds.

CASE CONTINUED

Height, weight, and head circumference are normal for his age. Upon further handling of the child, he exhibits a repetitive cluster of flexion contraction of the neck and trunk, with adduction and flexion of his arms and legs. A subsequent electroencephalogram (EEG) reveals a characteristic hypsarrhythmia pattern. The patient is diagnosed with infantile spasms.

Nonfebrile seizure disorders, or epilepsy, clinically represent abnormal neuronal discharge. Over 50% of cases are idiopathic. Some known causes include metabolic derangements, trauma, infections, neoplasms, toxins, and hereditary/genetic disorders. There are several conditions that can also mimic seizures such as tic disorders, reflux, breath-holding spells, syncope, tremor and other movement disorders, and benign positional vertigo.

QUESTIONS

89. Which of the following are types of generalized seizures?
    A. Absence
    B. Infantile spasms
    C. Tonic–clonic
    D. Atonic
    E. All of the above

90. Which statement about partial seizures is *incorrect*?
    A. Always involve impaired consciousness
    B. Can be associated with automatisms
    C. Can be characterized by a "Jacksonian march"
    D. May be preceded by an aura
    E. Is more common than generalized seizures

91. Which of following is *not* part of the initial management of status epilepticus?
    A. IV or rectal benzodiazepines
    B. ABC (airway, breathing, circulation) evaluation
    C. Assessment and correction of metabolic problems
    D. Assessment for underlying infection or trauma
    E. EEG

92. Which drug is inappropriately matched with its seizure type and common side effects?
    A. Ethosuximide: tonic–clonic/partial; associated with tremor and weight loss
    B. Valproic acid: tonic–clonic/partial; associated with hepatotoxicity, weight gain, and nausea
    C. Phenobarbital: tonic–clonic/partial; associated with hyperactivity, ataxia, and sedation
    D. Phenytoin: tonic–clonic/partial; associated with nystagmus and gum hyperplasia
    E. Carbamazepine: tonic–clonic/partial; associated with diplopia, blood dyscrasia, and ataxia

ID/CC: 14-year-old boy with crampy abdominal pain bloody diarrhea.

HPI: C.U. presents with abdominal pain and diarrhea that have been intermittent over the past several months. They are associated with fever, and diarrhea is occasionally bloody. The pain is not relieved by antacids, is mildly relieved by over-the-counter pain medications, and is not generally exacerbated by eating. He has had decreased appetite and energy levels during this period, and his mother notes a nearly 10-pound weight loss over the last year. He has no cough or rhinorrhea, no headache, and no noted trauma. The patient and his family are avid campers and traveled to South America last year, but no other members are ill nor are there any known ill contacts. His pain has been particularly bad over the last 2 days, with cramping in his lower abdomen.

PMHx:/PSHx: None **Meds:** As above **All:** NKDA **Immunizations:** UTD

SHx: Lives with mother, stepfather, and two younger siblings; no smokers, no pets. Not sexually active, no toxic habits, plays soccer and Sim City.

DietHx: Well-balanced diet, no particular foods seem to palliate or exacerbate symptoms, usually doesn't have "junk food."

VS: Temp 100.8°F, BP 100/55, HR 120, RR 24

PE: *Gen:* pale, alert, in no apparent distress. *HEENT:* NCAT, EOMI, normal exam *Neck:* supple. *Lungs:* normal exam. *CV:* mildly tachycardic, normal S_1, S_2, grade 1–2/6 systolic ejection murmur at left sternal border, pulses and cap refill normal. *Abdomen:* soft, nondistended, positive for right lower quadrant fullness/mass, positive bowel sounds, somewhat hypoactive, no HSM. *GU:* normal external male genitalia, Tanner stage 2.

THOUGHT QUESTIONS

- What is in your differential diagnosis?
- What further aspects of the physical examination or history will aid in the diagnosis?
- What diagnostic studies may aid you in your diagnosis?

For patients such as this, the differential diagnosis is quite extensive and can include infectious agents, hemolytic uremic syndrome, Henoch-Schönlein purpura, allergic colitis, lymphoma, inflammatory bowel disease, gynecologic causes (in females), appendicitis, and Meckel's diverticulum. Enteritis may be caused *Clostridium difficile, Campylobacter jejuni, Yersinia enterocolitica,* amebiasis, and *Giardia.* History and physical examination should include a thorough history of present illness, medications (antibiotics, chemotherapy agents), family history, review of growth curves, and a thorough review of systems. The physical examination should always include a rectal exam and inspection of the skin and extremities. Laboratory studies that may aid in making the diagnosis may include a CBC, stool studies (for toxins, ova and parasites, culture), protein markers, erythrocyte sedimentation rate (ESR), and imaging studies.

CASE CONTINUED

Further history reveals long-standing red and tender nodules that intermittently come and goes on his shins. He has also had transient knee pain over the last several weeks. A rectal exam reveals a skin tag on his perianal region, and yields positive guaiac results. The ESR was markedly elevated at 105; a CBC reveals a microcytic anemia; and albumin was low at 2. An upper GI study with small bowel follow-through showed narrowing at the terminal ileum (string sign). Contrast enema and subsequent endoscopy with biopsy confirmed the diagnosis of Crohn disease involvement of both the terminal ileum and large intestine, and management was initiated.

Inflammatory bowel disease (IBD) refers to two clinically distinct but related disorders: Crohn disease and ulcerative colitis (UC). In the pediatric population, they generally affect adolescents and are thought to be caused by a combination of genetic and environmental factors. Clinically, ulcerative colitis generally tends to present with symptoms affecting the large intestine, whereas Crohn disease may affect any part of the GI tract. Both can be associated with fever, weight loss, and poor growth. Laboratory studies may show anemia and decreased serum protein markers. Contrast enema studies as well as upper GI contrast studies can aid in the diagnosis. Endoscopy and biopsy generally confirm the diagnosis. The nodules on the lower extremities in this patient were indicative of erythema nodosum, which can be associated with Crohn disease.

QUESTIONS

93. Which is least likely to be an extraintestinal manifestation of IBD?
    A. Arthritis
    B. Anterior uveitis
    C. Aphthous ulcers
    D. Acanthosis nigricans
    E. Ankylosing spondylitis

94. Which of the following is more common with Crohn's disease as compared to ulcerative colitis?
    A. Transmural involvement
    B. Almost always involves the rectum
    C. Restricted to large intestine
    D. Crypt abscesses
    E. Higher risk for developing cancer

95. Which of the following are not commonly involved in IBD therapy?
    A. Corticosteroids
    B. Sulfasalazine
    C. Surgery
    D. Nutritional support
    E. Metoclopramide

96. Which of the following statements about IBD are *false*?
    A. Crohn patients may present with an abdominal mass.
    B. Ulcerative colitis can be complicated by toxic megacolon.
    C. Fistula formation rarely occurs.
    D. Nutrient loss is common.
    E. It may involve delayed sexual development.

ID/CC: 4-year-old girl with watery diarrhea over the past 6 days presents to urgent care clinic with lethargy.

HPI: D.D. was in her usual state of good health until 1 week ago when she awoke twice in the middle of the night with diarrhea. She had just returned the night before from a family vacation to South America. The diarrhea was clear, watery, and with no blood. She complained of crampy abdominal pain occurring just prior to each watery stool. The diarrhea has continued throughout the week, occurring 3 to 4 times daily, and she has been afebrile. She has not been able to keep any foods or liquids down for at least the past 2 days, and her mother is concerned that she has appeared very weak since this morning. She has also not urinated since yesterday morning. Fortunately she has not had any seizures, but her mental status has changed slightly today accompanied by an increasingly tired appearance. Her mother was very careful about not letting her eat or drink suspicious foods during their trip, but does remember the girl adding some ice to her Coke at the airport cafeteria just before they left to return home. She has lost about 3 to 4 pounds over the past week (her last recorded weight was 30 pounds).

THOUGHT QUESTIONS

- What is in this patient's differential diagnosis?
- What is the significance of the weakness and lethargy?

The differential diagnosis of acute diarrhea includes infectious causes (e.g., viral gastroenteritis, bacterial enterocolitis, hepatitis, food poisoning, otitis media, UTI); GI causes (e.g., intussusception, appendicitis); toxic ingestions (e.g., salicylates, lead); renal causes (e.g., hemolytic uremic syndrome); and vasculitis (e.g., Henoch-Schönlein purpura). The most common causes of watery diarrhea are endotoxin-mediated and are caused by *Escherichia coli* and *Vibrio cholerae*.

Weakness and lethargy in the face of a decreased urine output and weight loss indicates that this patient is probably suffering from dehydration. If she were also having any evidence of seizures or high fevers accompanied by behavioral changes, additional explanations for lethargy could include sepsis (e.g., meningitis, encephalitis) or toxic ingestions.

CASE CONTINUED

PMHx:/PSHx: None   **Meds:** None   **All:** NKDA

FHx: No history of inflammatory bowel disorders.

SHx: Lives at home with mother and father. Attends daycare 5 times a week.

VS: Temp 100.5°F, BP 88/62, HR 90, RR 28

PE: *Gen:* awake, alert, crying (no tears). *HEENT:* mucous membranes dry, eyes mildly sunken, throat nonerythematous. *Lungs:* clear bilaterally. *Abdomen:* soft, nondistended, minimal tenderness to touch especially over stomach, otherwise no guarding; positive bowel sounds, no masses. *Skin:* capillary refill time 3 sec.

THOUGHT QUESTION

- In addition to physical examination, what three laboratory tests are helpful in determining the degree of dehydration?

In general, an arterial blood gas, serum electrolyte panel (including BUN), and urine specific gravity may be helpful in determining the degree of dehydration. A marked base deficit on ABG may reflect metabolic acidosis secondary to poor perfusion from dehydration. The BUN may be elevated secondary to a hemoconcentrating effect; similarly, an elevated urine specific gravity indicates a concentrated urine from decreased excretion of water.

Labs: Electrolytes (mEq/L): Na 135, K 4, Cl 100, HCO_3 22, BUN 35, creatinine 0.8, ABG: pH 7.29, pCO_2 35, PaO_2 85, B.E. −5, Urine spec grav 1.025.

QUESTIONS

97. Which of the following clinical manifestations of dehydration is the last to develop?
    A. Tachycardia
    B. Weight loss
    C. Decreased urine output
    D. Hypotension
    E. No tears when crying

98. Based on the physical exam of the patient presented in this case scenario, an estimate of her degree of dehydration is:
    A. She is not dehydrated.
    B. Mild dehydration
    C. Moderate dehydration
    D. Severe dehydration

99. The patient presented in this case scenario most likely has which type of dehydration?
    A. Hypotonic
    B. Hyponatremic
    C. Isotonic
    D. Hypertonic

100. During replacement therapy for dehydration, most deficits are replaced over 24 hours, with half given over the first 8 hours and half over the next 16 hours. The exception is hypertonic dehydration, in which the deficit is replaced slowly over 48 to 72 hours to prevent:
    A. Hypertension
    B. Tachycardia
    C. Brain edema
    D. Hydrocephalus

ID/CC: 3-year-old girl with vomiting and diarrhea over the past 2 days presents to urgent care clinic in the afternoon.

HPI: V.G. was in her usual state of good health until 2 nights ago when she awoke twice in the middle of the night with vomiting. The vomitus was clear, nonbilious fluid with no blood. She had eaten a meal of macaroni and cheese which her 9-year-old brother had also eaten; he subsequently slept without difficulty. Her mother remembers that a friend of the little girl's from daycare also had a similar vomiting bout a week earlier, which resolved on its own. She complained of crampy abdominal pain just prior to the vomiting with no pain in between. By the next evening she began to have clear diarrhea (no blood) occurring 3 to 4 times throughout the day which was accompanied by a low-grade fever. Today she has not been able to keep any foods or liquids down and last urinated this morning.

THOUGHT QUESTIONS

- What is in this patient's differential diagnosis?
- What is the significance of bilious vomiting, if present?

The differential diagnosis of acute vomiting and diarrhea is extensive and includes infectious causes (e.g., viral, bacterial enterocolitis, hepatitis, food poisoning, peritonitis, pharyngitis, pneumonia, otitis media, tonsillitis, UTI); metabolic causes (e.g., diabetic ketoacidosis, adrenal crisis, renal or hepatic failure), central nervous system causes (i.e., increased intracranial pressure, meningitis, encephalitis, labyrinthitis, migraine, Reye syndrome, seizure, tumor), GI causes (e.g., appendicitis, bowel obstruction); respiratory causes (e.g., reactive airways disease), and toxic ingestions (e.g., salicylates, lead).

The significance of bilious vomiting in any patient indicates a complete or partial obstructive process and almost always warrants corrective or exploratory surgical intervention.

PMHx/PSHx: None   **Meds:** None   **All:** NKDA

FHx: No history of inflammatory bowel disorders.

SHx: Lives at home with mother, father and 9-year-old brother. Attends daycare 2 times a week.

VS: Temp 100.5°F, BP 88/62, HR 79, RR 28

PE: *Gen:* awake, alert, crying (with tears). *HEENT:* mucous membranes dry, throat nonerythematous. *Lungs:* clear bilaterally. *Abdomen:* soft, nondistended, minimal tenderness to touch especially over stomach; otherwise no guarding; positive bowel sounds, no masses. *Skin:* well-perfused, capillary refill time <2 sec.

THOUGHT QUESTIONS

- What laboratory tests, if any, are appropriate to obtain at this time?
- What is the most important aspect of the physical examination that will determine the aggressiveness of therapy?

In general, if an infectious agent is considered, only a CBC with blood culture need be obtained. If a strong suspicion of viral gastroenteritis is made, it is acceptable to perform no laboratory tests, provided the patient's fluid status is in balance.

The most important assessment of the physical examination is to determine the patient's hydration status. A moderate to severely dehydrated child may need more aggressive intervention to rehydrate.

Labs: CBC: WBC 18,000; 2% bands, 20% neut, 30% lymphocytes.

CASE CONTINUED

Given the low-grade fever and the history of ill contact a week prior, you determine the most likely cause of this patient's vomiting and diarrhea is viral gastroenteritis.

QUESTIONS

101. The agent most likely to cause acute gastroenteritis is:
    A. *Staphylococcus aureus*
    B. *Clostridium perfringens*
    C. Rotavirus
    D. *Escherichia coli*
    E. Adenovirus

102. The most appropriate treatment for a mildly dehydrated child with acute gastroenteritis is:
    A. Surgical laparotomy
    B. Admit to hospital for IV fluids
    C. Admit to hospital for IV fluids followed by inpatient oral rehydration
    D. Admit to hospital for IV fluids followed by outpatient oral rehydration
    E. Outpatient oral rehydration

103. The most common cause of parasitic watery diarrhea in the U.S. is:
    A. *Entamoeba histolytica*
    B. *Giardia lamblia*
    C. Schistosomiasis
    D. *Ascaris lumbricoides*

104. The toxin associated with a history of antibiotic overuse is:
    A. *E. coli*
    B. *Yersinia enterocolitica*
    C. *Clostridium difficile*
    D. *Clostridium perfringens*
    E. *Giardia lamblia*

ID/CC: 5-week-old baby boy presents to urgent care clinic with vomiting for past 2 weeks.

HPI: P.S. was born at full term (38 weeks' GA) by NSVD to a 26-year-old woman, G1, P1, A+, serology (–), rubella immune, hepatitis B (–), VDRL (–), who had good prenatal care. She had a routine 20-week prenatal sonogram that revealed a normal fetus and amniotic fluid. At delivery, baby P.S. was vigorous, with Apgar scores of 9 and 9, and a birth weight of 2780 gram. He was discharged to home breastfeeding well 2 days after delivery and had a normal 2-week visit at which time his weight was noted to be 2790 gram with a normal physical examination. His mother states that for the past 2 weeks he has been having increasing spitting up, and recently over the last 3 days has had very force-ful vomiting described as "projectile" in nature. He has been breastfed every 3 to 4 hours and his mother feels he has a good suck and swallow. He had a normal stooling pattern with four stools per day of mustard yellow and seedy consistency, although he has had only one such stool in the last 3 days. He now feeds for only about 5 minutes per breast and vomits most of the quantity within 10 minutes. Today his weight is still 2790 gram.

THOUGHT QUESTIONS

- What is in this patient's differential diagnosis?
- What is the significance of today's weight?

The differential diagnosis of a newborn infant with vomiting can be divided into two categories: bilious and nonbilious. Bilious vomiting generally involves conditions with partial or complete bowel obstruction such as malrotation, volvulus, Ladd's bands, Hirschsprung disease, incarcerated hernia, torsion of Meckel's diverticulum and intestinal atresia. Nonbilious vomiting in a newborn is largely due to gastroesophageal reflux, cow or soy milk protein intolerance, and pyloric stenosis. Although rare, nonbilious vomiting may also occur in esophageal atresia, but is usually diagnosed immediately after initiation of feeds.

The significance of today's weight is that there has been no growth since the patient's last visit nearly 3 weeks ago. In general, babies gain weight at an average of about 20 gram per day. Thus, this infant's weight should have been closer to 3200 grams. The poor weight gain points to a definite pathological cause associated with the vomiting history.

PMHx/PSHx: None **Meds:** None **All:** NKDA

FHx: Baby's mother reports having had a surgical procedure because of vomiting when she was an infant.

SHx: Lives at home with mother and father. At home with mother during the day.

VS: Temp 98.5°F, BP 88/62, HR 79, RR 28

PE: *Gen:* awake, alert, crying (no tears). *HEENT:* mucous membranes dry, eyes mildly sunken, throat nonerythematous. *Lungs:* Clear bilaterally. *Abdomen:* soft, nondistended; positive bowel sounds, small 3- to 4-cm "olive" sized slightly firm round mass felt just to the right of the umbilicus. *Skin:* well-perfused.

THOUGHT QUESTION

- What radiologic test would be helpful at this time?

An abdominal ultrasound can help to confirm the diagnosis of pyloric stenosis, showing a thickened ring in the region of the pylorus. Rarely, an upper GI contrast series can also be performed, but is usually not necessary if the history, physical examination, and ultrasound are confirmatory.

CASE CONTINUED

You determine this baby has pyloric stenosis. The most important next step is to determine the patient's hydration status. From the physical examination you note that he must be at least mildly to moderately dehydrated and decide to correct his fluid status before consulting the pediatric surgeons for corrective surgical repair.

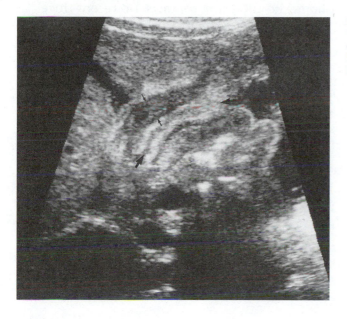

FIGURE 27 Ultrasound of a baby with pyloric stenosis. Arrows indicate the elongated pyloric canal (*thick arrow*) and thickened pyloric muscle (*thin arrows*). Used with permission from Rudolf M, Levene Paediatrics and Child Health. Oxford: Blackwell Science, Ltd., 1999: 160.

QUESTIONS

105. Additional findings associated with pyloric stenosis can often include:
    A. Simian crease
    B. Visible gastric peristaltic waves
    C. A "double bubble" sign on abdominal x-ray
    D. Bloody stools

106. The most common condition requiring surgery in the first 2 months of life for term newborn infants is:
    A. Inguinal hernia
    B. Pyloric stenosis
    C. Cardiac atrioventricular canal defect
    D. Malrotation of the intestines

107. The surgical treatment of choice for pyloric stenosis is:
    A. Nissen fundoplication
    B. Esophagomyotomy
    C. Pyloric resection
    D. Pyloromyotomy

108. The metabolic derangement often associated with pyloric stenosis is:
    A. Hyperkalemic metabolic acidosis
    B. Hyperkalemic metabolic alkalosis
    C. Hypokalemic metabolic acidosis
    D. Hypokalemic metabolic alkalosis

ID/CC: 18-month-old boy with intermittent emesis and irritability.

HPI: B.I. was well prior to 2 days ago when mother noticed he had bouts of irritability and vomiting. Mother states that the vomiting is nonbloody and nonbilious, and "he seems to be cramping in pain." The episodes seem to be interspersed with periods of normal behavior and feeding, but she is more worried today as they have increased in frequency and he is looking more tired. He does not have any cough or runny nose, nor does he have any rash. He had just recovered from a "cold" last week and was otherwise well. He has had a slight temperature today. Mother tried giving acetaminophen without any resolve.

PMHx:/PSHx: None **Meds:** Tylenol as above

SHx: Lives with mother and father, older sibling at home; no current ill contacts. No recent travel.

FHx: None

VS: Temp 100.5°F, BP 110/65, HR 160, RR 26

PE: *Gen:* child is interactive with mother but appears tired and lethargic. Dry oral mucous membranes, decreased skin turgor. *Lungs:* clear to auscultation. *CV:* tachycardic, but with no murmur, capillary refill time is nearly 3 sec. *Abdomen:* distended, tympanic but soft, no visceromegaly, soft palpable mass in right upper quadrant, hypoactive bowel sounds.

THOUGHT QUESTIONS

- What further history may be helpful?
- What further physical examination findings may be helpful?
- What is included in the differential diagnosis?
- What studies would be appropriate for narrowing your diagnosis?

In particular, further questions regarding the bowel history are likely to contribute to the diagnosis with either positive or negative responses. These questions include frequency, quantity, concomitant symptoms, whether the patient has diarrhea and whether the stools are bloody. The physical examination for any patient with GI complaints should include a rectal exam and a guaiac performed to test for occult blood. The differential diagnosis for this patient includes acute gastroenteritis, causes of intestinal obstruction, appendicitis, malrotation, Meckel's diverticula, and abdominal wall herniation. To further elucidate the diagnosis, plain films of the abdomen including a KUB and upright can provide information in the setting of obstruction and intussusception. If appendicitis is suspected, spiral CT is most commonly used to confirm diagnosis.

CASE CONTINUED

Further questioning of the parent reveals a history of rectal bleeding at home. Rectal exam performed during the physical examination has confirmed this. A plain film of the abdomen revealed distended bowel loops and air-fluid levels. A subsequent air-contrast enema revealed a "coiled-spring" appearance to the small bowel and an ileocolic intussusception.

Intussusception results from the telescoping of a portion of proximal bowel into adjacent distal bowel. Most commonly this is an ileocolic process. Compression of the bowel wall and obstruction of blood supply lead to ischemia and infarction. If untreated, the results can be disastrous, leading to abdominal distention, perforation, and shock. The classic triad is a history of brief, colicky, intermittent bouts of abdominal pain every 5 to 30 minutes, vomiting, and bloody stools.

QUESTIONS

109. Which of the following is *not* generally considered to be a "lead point" for intussusception?
    A. Meckel's diverticulum
    B. Hypertrophied Peyer's patch
    C. Lymphoma
    D. Duodenal ulcer
    E. Foreign body

110. Abdominal exam of a patient with intussusception is *not* likely to reveal which of the following?
    A. Sausage-shaped mass in right side
    B. Abdominal distention
    C. Hepatosplenomegaly
    D. Normal findings
    E. Peritoneal signs

111. Which of the following statements about intussusception is *true*?
    A. Usually affects patients after age 3.
    B. The majority are unsuccessfully reduced via pneumatic or hydrostatic methods.
    C. Cause is unknown in the majority of cases.
    D. IV hydration and nasogastric decompression are generally not indicated.
    E. There is virtually no recurrence after reduction.

112. Which of the following is *not* commonly included in the differential diagnosis for acute abdominal pain?
    A. Acute viral gastroenteritis
    B. Food poisoning
    C. Food allergy
    D. Bacterial enterocolitis
    E. Obstructive bowel disease

ID/CC: 4-year-old boy brought in by his father after he vomited blood in daycare today.

HPI: N.B. was in his usual good state of health this morning when he left for daycare. He has not had any recent illnesses or vomiting, although he tends to have a "sensitive stomach." Today he was playing at school when he suddenly ran to the bathroom to throw up. The teacher noticed that there were some small brownish clots in the vomitus, and called his father to pick him up. N.B. has not been complaining of abdominal pain, has been eating and drinking normally, and stooling normally. He has not vomited since this morning, and seems to feel "fine" though he is somewhat fearful.

PMHx: No hospitalizations, no surgeries. Allergic rhinitis, uses nasal steroids for control.

Meds: None; no recent use of NSAIDs   **All:** NKDA   **Immunization:** UTD

FHx: Negative for hematologic disorders, peptic ulcer or liver disease.

THOUGHT QUESTIONS

- What is your first concern with this patient?
- What are possible sources of the bleeding?

In any patient that has evidence of GI bleeding, you should initially be concerned with the patient's hemodynamic stability. Perform a brief physical survey and check the patient's vital signs for tachycardia, an early sign of volume depletion in children. After confirming that the patient is stable, try to establish whether the substance is actually blood. Use the appropriate test depending on the body fluid being tested (i.e., Gastroccult for emesis, Hemoccult for stool). Finally, think about where the bleeding is coming from, and whether it is continuing. In the case of an upper GI bleed, consider gastric lavage with warm saline to look for a persistent bleeding source.

Bleeding from the GI tract should be characterized as from either an upper or a lower GI source. An upper GI bleed, one that occurs proximal to the ligament of Treitz, presents as bright red or "coffee ground" emesis. Conversely, a lower GI bleed presents as bright red blood per rectum or in stool. Melena or heme positive stool can signify either an upper or a lower source, so a nasogastric aspirate should be obtained to confirm the location. In this case, you are concerned about an upper GI bleed, so any of the structures proximal to the ligament of Treitz (i.e., duodenal bulb, stomach, esophagus, oropharynx, and nose) can be responsible. Additional exam and history should be directed toward establishing a history of disease or trauma involving these structures.

CASE CONTINUED

You check the patient's vital signs, which reveal a temperature of 37.0°C (98.6°F), pulse of 85, respiratory rate of 21, and blood pressure of 105/70. Feeling reassured that your patient is hemodynamically stable, you obtain further history and perform a careful physical examination. You call the teacher at the daycare to confirm that no sharp objects could have been ingested, and elicit an additional piece of information: N.B. had a nosebleed that morning prior to the vomiting. The teacher reports that the nosebleed stopped after 5 minutes of direct pressure, and N.B. went back to playing afterward. You confirm with the family that there is no history of NSAID use or of bruising or bleeding prior to this episode. The parents mention that N.B. has nosebleeds about once a week, and that they always stop promptly.

PE: *Gen:* reveals a well-appearing boy with a nasal voice. *HEENT:* right nares is crusted with blood, left is normal. *CV:* RR&R, no murmur, pulses and cap refill brisk. *Abdomen:* soft, nondistended and nontender, normoactive bowel sounds, no masses. *Skin:* pink and warm, no bruising or petechiae.

Reassured by your further history and the physical examination, and given the new piece of history, you decide that N.B. probably vomited blood after epistaxis. The most common reason for epistaxis in children is nose picking, but in this case N.B. has two additional risk factors: allergic rhinitis and the use of nasal steroids. You discuss these findings with the parents and suggest that they discontinue the nasal steroids, use an oral antihistamine instead, and apply a lubricant to the nose to combat dryness. With careful follow-up, N.B. has no further episodes of hematemesis, and his nosebleeds improve on the new allergy regimen.

QUESTIONS

113. Bright red blood per rectum is likely to be caused by each of the following *except*:
    A. Peptic ulcer disease
    B. Ulcerative colitis
    C. Anal fissure
    D. Constipation

114. In a patient with an active upper GI bleed you should:
    A Perform gastric lavage with warm saline solution.
    B. Initiate fluid resuscitation.
    C. Send blood for CBC, type and crossmatch.
    D. Do all of the above.

115. Which of the following is *true* of Meckel's diverticulum?
    A. It usually presents as painful rectal bleeding.
    B. It is a relatively uncommon anomaly of the GI tract.
    C. It is usually composed of heterotopic gastric tissue.
    D. The peak incidence of bleeding is in early adolescence.

116. Which of the following is *true* concerning GI bleeds in children?
    A. Upper GI bleeds are more common than lower GI bleeds.
    B. Melena is always caused by blood.
    C. Rectal bleeding is an uncommon presentation.
    D. The differential diagnosis varies based on age.

ID/CC: 8-year-old girl presents to emergency room at 7 AM complaining of pain in left leg during walking.

HPI: T.S. was in her usual state of good health until yesterday morning when she noticed slight pain in her left thigh occasionally when she walked. The pain had become slightly worse throughout the day but she was able to sleep through the night. The pain is worse this morning. She insists the leg hurts only when she walks or tries to run, and reports no history of recent trauma to her leg (especially as her mother did not allow her to play in her soccer league last week because she still had a cold). She describes the pain as being "dull" with a gradual onset and feels it mostly in her hip. It is worsened by bearing weight and improves slightly when she rests.

PMHx:/PSHx: Normal weight gain   **Meds:** Tylenol PRN for pain   **All:** NKDA

FHx: No history of familial orthopedic, endocrine, or oncologic disorders.

SHx: Lives at home with her mother, father, and older brother aged 12. Attends 2nd grade and is currently in a local girls' soccer league.

VS: Temp 98.8°F, BP 95/68, HR 74, RR 22

PE: *Gen:* awake, alert and oriented × 3. *Ext:* left leg is well perfused. No visible bleeding, bruising, or joint swelling noted. Normal range of motion of knee and ankle, but guarding of hip on internal rotation. No pain on palpation except pain at hip while standing. Normal sensory exam and proprioception of leg. Unable to walk due to pain. Remainder of physical exam normal.

THOUGHT QUESTIONS

- What is in this patient's differential diagnosis?
- What three hematologic laboratory tests should be obtained at this time?
- What is the significance of the history of a recent cold?
- Although x-rays may also be helpful, what single procedure may yield a definitive diagnosis?

This patient's differential diagnosis mainly includes traumatic injury, infectious causes such as toxic synovitis, early septic arthritis or osteomyelitis, rheumatologic disease, and, less likely, malignancy.

With this broad differential, laboratory tests should be geared toward identifying the presence of infection or inflammation, which will help to narrow the possibilities and guide further investigation. The hematologic tests to order at this time are CBC with differential, ESR, and blood culture.

The significance of the recent cold is that it may suggest toxic synovitis, an inflammatory postinfectious arthritis that is commonly preceded by an upper respiratory viral infection.

Whenever septic arthritis is a possibility, aspiration of joint fluid is the definitive test that should be performed to confirm or eliminate this diagnosis. X-rays can be helpful to differentiate between transient toxic synovitis or septic arthritis versus osteomyelitis. In some cases of septic arthritis, there may be a notable widening of the space between the femoral head and acetabulum. Malignancies or osteomyelitis may also be detected on x-ray by irregularities or lucencies in the bone, although these findings are usually delayed by 5 or more days. Other imaging studies that are useful for examining bones and joints include MRI and bone scan. These should be considered on a case-by-case basis.

CASE CONTINUED

Labs: WBC 18,000 (60% lymphs, 25% segs, 0 bands); ESR 22. Blood culture in lab. X-ray left leg: normal. No increase in joint space of left hip. No lucencies.

Based on the patient's well appearance, absence of findings on x-ray or on examination consistent with a septic joint, and reassuring laboratory studies, you determine the patient has toxic synovitis.

QUESTIONS

117. Management of toxic synovitis includes all of the following *except*:
     A. Rest
     B. Anti-inflammatory medications
     C. Antibiotics
     D. Close follow-up exams

118. If this patient had high fevers, significantly elevated WBC, ESR >25, positive finding of increased joint space on hip x-ray, and purulent fluid from joint aspiration, the next step would be:
     A. Ask patient to return next day for repeat WBC and ESR
     B. Open joint drainage and initiation of IV antibiotics
     C. IV antibiotics only
     D. Oral antibiotics only
     E. Bone scan

119. The most common organism causing septic arthritis in a patient with sickle cell disease is:
     A. *Salmonella typhi*
     B. *Haemophilus influenzae* type B
     C. *Staphylococcus aureus*
     D. *Streptococcus pneumoniae*
     E. *Neisseria gonorrhoeae*

120. The most common cause of monoarthritis or polyarthritis in an adolescent is:
     A. *Salmonella typhi*
     B. *Haemophilus influenzae* type B
     C. *Staphylococcus aureus*
     D. *Streptococcus pneumoniae*
     E. *Neisseria gonorrhoeae*

ID/CC: 11-year-old girl with fever presents to pediatric urgent care clinic with left knee pain.

HPI: R.A. was in her usual state of health until 6 weeks ago when she began to have intermittent low-grade fevers and joint swelling of her left knee. She does not remember any trauma to the leg and has not had any intercurrent viral illness. When asked about the quality of the pain, she states it is "dull," constant, limited to her knee and hurts more at night. It is so uncomfortable that she has been limping for 2 days. Her only other symptoms include feeling tired and a slight loss of appetite. She denies any recent trips into the woods and is not sexually active.

PMHx:/PSHx: None   **Meds:** None   **All:** NKDA

FHx: Mother has (systemic lupus erythematosus) SLE. No oncologic disorders.

SHx: Lives at home with mother and father; attends 5th grade.

VS: Temp 100.5°F, BP 105/72, HR 79, RR 28

PE: *Gen:* awake, alert and oriented × 3. *HEENT:* normal. *Neck:* positive lymphadenopathy (bilateral anterior cervical). *Abdomen:* positive hepatosplenomegaly. *Ext:* left leg: swelling of knee joint. No erythema but slightly warm. Decreased range of motion and minimal pain on palpation. Remainder of exam normal.

THOUGHT QUESTIONS

• What is in this patient's differential diagnosis?

• What are at least two antibody titers that are worth obtaining?

The differential diagnosis of an isolated arthritis includes juvenile rheumatoid arthritis (JRA), systemic lupus erythematosus (SLE), septic arthritis with or without osteomyelitis, toxic synovitis, Lyme disease, and residual inflammation following injury. The significance of the lymphadenopathy and hepatosplenomegaly in this case points more toward a systemic condition.

Antibody tests that are worth ordering are an acetylneuraminic acid (ANA) and RF, in addition to a CBC, ESR, and blood culture. The ANA is a sensitive but nonspecific test for many autoimmune diseases, including SLE, dermatomyositis, and JRA. RF is usually negative in children with JRA, but if positive is associated with more severe prognosis and with ophthalmologic disease.

CASE CONTINUED

Labs: (+) ANA, (–) RF. WBC 15,000, Hb 11 g/dL, plts 298,000, ESR 30. X-ray: left knee: No lucencies, no bony abnormalities, slight suggestion of joint soft tissue swelling.

You determine this patient must have a form of JRA, most likely a pauciarticular form, as compared to polyarticular or systemic disease. She does not have polyarticular disease because she has less than five or more affected joints, and does not have systemic disease because she did not exhibit temperature elevations greater than 103°F for 2 weeks, no rash, and minimal ESR elevation.

TABLE 31. Classification of Juvenile Rheumatoid Arthritis

	POLYARTHRITIS	OLIGOARTHRITIS	SYSTEMIC
Total cases (%)	40–50	40–50	10–20
Number, pattern of joints involved	≥5; symmetric	≤4; may be only a single joint	Variable
Type of joints involved	Large (knees, elbows, ankles, wrists) and cervical joints	Knees and/or ankles	Any joint
Severity of systemic involvement	Moderate	Rare	Severe[a]
Development of chronic uveitis (%)	5	20	Rare
Rh factor (+) (%)	10	Rare	Rare
ANA factor (+) (%)	50	80	10

[a]Including a high, spiking fever one to two times a day and a characteristic rheumatoid rash (erythematous macules on trunk, extremities) lasting over 1 hour.

Modified from Cassidy JT. Connective tissue diseases and amyloidosis. In: Oski FA, DeAngelis CD, Feigin FD, et al., eds. Principles and Practice of Pediatrics, 2nd ed. Philadelphia: J.B. Lippincott Company, 1994: 246.

QUESTIONS

121. This patient does not have SLE because:
    A. SLE does not run in families.
    B. She has a positive ANA titer.
    C. She has a negative RF titer.
    D. She does not meet at least 4 of the 11 clinical criteria to diagnose SLE.

122. This patient may eventually develop all of the following *except*:
    A. Uveitis
    B. Ankylosing spondylitis
    C. Polyarteritis nodosa
    D. Reiter syndrome

123. Which of the following statements regarding resolution of JRA is *true*?
    A. 20% of all children with JRA will "outgrow" their disease.
    B. 40% of all children with JRA will "outgrow" their disease.
    C. 60% of all children with JRA will "outgrow" their disease.
    D. 80% of all children with JRA will "outgrow" their disease.

124. Which of the following statements regarding JRA is *false*?
    A. Morning stiffness is a characteristic complaint.
    B. Pain symptoms are variable.
    C. Generalized growth retardation may occur.
    D. X-ray changes in JRA are usually severe.

ID/CC: 4-year-old boy presents to the pediatric urgent care clinic at noon complaining of pain in his right shoulder.

HPI: The mother says she picked up N.E. from daycare after she received a call that he was crying and had fallen during a game of tug-of-war (his team lost). When asked what had happened, the boy simply said he got pulled "hard" by the rope and fell into the sandbox. When asked where it hurt, the boy used his left hand and pointed up and down his right upper arm, keeping it still. He is not able to answer specific questions about the quality of the pain (sharp vs. dull, intermittent or constant), because he always just answers "yes." His mother reports that she has not seen him move his arm since she picked him up, and that he was in good health when he awoke this morning and has had no previous history of injuries to his right arm.

PMHx:/PSHx: None   **Meds:** None   **All:** NKDA

FHx: No history of familial orthopedic or connective tissue disorders.

SHx: Lives at home with his mother and father. No siblings. Attends daycare 3 days a week.

VS: Temp 98.4°F, BP 90/60, HR 80, RR 28

PE: *Gen:* awake, alert. *Ext:* right arm: held at side, slightly flexed and pronated. No bleeding, bruising, or lacerations. No visible swelling of shoulder, elbow, or wrist joints. No pain on palpation of shoulder, elbow, or wrist joints. No pain on palpation of the humerus or bones of the arm or wrist. The boy refuses to straighten the arm or use it to reach for objects. Remainder of exam was within normal limits.

THOUGHT QUESTIONS

- What is in this patient's differential diagnosis?
- What would be the next diagnostic test?
- How does isolation of pain relate to true location of injury in limb injuries?
- What is the significance, if any, about the position of the patient's arm?

The differential diagnosis primarily includes acute traumatic conditions: fracture of the wrist or arm bones, dislocation of the shoulder, or subluxation of the radial head (nursemaid's elbow). Occasionally an infectious or malignant process in the bone or joint can come to the parent or child's attention after trauma, so these possibilities should be kept in mind as well. Fractures in children require special attention, especially if they extend through the epiphyseal growth plate. (See Figure 32.)

The next diagnostic test to perform is x-ray of right arm to rule out fractures. It is important to include standard and oblique views of shoulder, elbow, and wrist, because an injury in any of these locations can cause this child's symptoms.

The concept of "referred" pain in limb injuries is important to consider, because a child may perceive and thus point to an area and complain of pain even when the actual injury site is elsewhere.

The slightly flexed and pronated position of the patient's arm at his side strongly suggests subluxation of the radial head (nursemaid's elbow). Additionally, lack of point tenderness on palpation is less consistent with fracture (although, rarely, some fractures may not be immediately associated with pain).

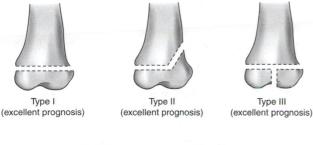

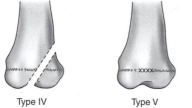

Type I
(excellent prognosis)

Type II
(excellent prognosis)

Type III
(excellent prognosis)

Type IV

Type V

(high risk for growth disturbance)

FIGURE 32 Epiphyseal fractures: Salter-Harris classification. Illustration by Electronic Illustrators Group.

CASE CONTINUED

Labs: X-ray right arm: no fracture or soft-tissue swelling noted.

Based on the typical history and physical examination, and negative chest x-ray, you determine this patient's injury must be a subluxation of the radial head (nursemaid's elbow).

QUESTIONS

125. Treatment of nursemaid's elbow consists of applying pressure on the radial head and:
    A. Holding elbow in full extension and manipulating forearm into pronation
    B. Holding elbow in full extension and manipulating forearm into supination
    C. Holding elbow in 90° flexion and manipulating forearm into pronation
    D. Holding elbow in 90° flexion and manipulating forearm into supination
    E. Consulting an orthopedic surgeon

126. When nursemaid's elbow is suspected, the patient:
    A. Is unable to move the extremity
    B. Is able to pronate and supinate forearm
    C. Can only supinate forearm
    D. Is unable to flex or extend forearm
    E. Can slightly flex or extend forearm

127. Recurrent subluxation of the radial head should be treated:
    A. Conservatively with no treatment
    B. By splinting the arm for 2 weeks
    C. By casting the arm for 2 weeks
    D. By surgical pinning of the radial head to the ulna

128. Which of the following statements regarding dislocated shoulders is *true*?
    A. It occurs more commonly in infants.
    B. It occurs more commonly in toddlers.
    C. It occurs more commonly in adolescents. It occurs with the same frequency throughout childhood (infants to adolescents).

ID/CC: 6-month-old African American infant presents to urgent care clinic with painful swollen hands and feet.

HPI: S.A. was brought to clinic by a caretaker from his foster home when she noted that he awoke this morning and appeared to have slight swelling of his hands and feet. Over the course of the morning, he has become increasingly irritable and the swelling has worsened. He immediately cries when his hands or feet are touched. He has been afebrile and has not had any ill contacts. His birth history is unknown because he was abandoned at birth by his mother and left in a blanket on the doorstep of an inner-city orphanage. He was in good health when he was found, has not had any illnesses to date, and has had excellent weight gain since birth. He was well until this morning with no signs of respiratory infections, no vomiting, diarrhea, other rashes or bruising, and no reported history of trauma. He is developmentally normal.

PMHx:/PSHx: None **Meds:** None **All:** NKDA **FHx:** Unknown.

SHx: Lives in a foster home since age 2 months with his adoptive mother and father, both healthy. No pets. His adoptive mother stays home with him during the day.

VS: Temp 97°F, BP 80/65, HR 100, RR 40

PE: *Gen:* awake, alert, fussy. Cries when hands or feet are touched. *HEENT:* normocephalic, ant. fontanel soft/flat. Eyes PERRLA, normal fundi, normal ears. *Lungs:* clear bilaterally. *CV:* RR&R, normal S_1, S_2, slight flow murmur heard over entire chest. *Abdomen:* soft, nondistended, positive bowel sounds, no masses, normal liver edge. Palpable spleen tip in left upper quadrant. *Ext:* both hands and feet slightly warm to touch with marked swelling mostly over dorsum. *Skin:* no rashes, cyanosis, bruising, or wounds.

THOUGHT QUESTIONS
- What is in this patient's differential diagnosis?
- What is the significance of a palpable spleen tip?

This patient's differential diagnosis includes sickle cell disease, trauma, osteomyelitis, juvenile rheumatoid arthritis (JRA), and tumors of bones. Because he is affected bilaterally and symmetrically in the upper and lower extremities, the most likely diagnosis is a more generalized process such as sickle cell disease.

The significance of a palpable spleen tip indicates an enlarged spleen. In sickle cell disease, splenic enlargement occurs as a result of sequestration crisis in which the spleen suddenly becomes engorged with red blood cells, trapping a significant portion of the blood volume.

Labs: CBC: WBC 15,000; Hb 6 g/dL, Hct 20, plts 150. No bands on differential. X-rays of hands and feet: marked soft tissue swelling, no fractures.

CASE CONTINUED

You determine this patient has presented with dactylitis secondary to sickle cell disease and admit the child to the hospital to initiate appropriate hydration therapy and pain medication.

QUESTIONS

129. The diagnosis of sickle cell disease can be made by all of the following, *except*:
    A. Newborn screening tests (in most states)
    B. Hemoglobin electrophoresis
    C. Splenic ultrasound
    D. Sickledex preparation to demonstrate sickling of red blood cells at low O_2 tension

130. Which of the following combinations of quantitative hemoglobin electrophoresis is characteristic of sickle cell trait?
    A. 0% hemoglobin A, 2% to 3% hemoglobin A2, 85% to 95% hemoglobin S, 5% to 15% hemoglobin F
    B. 55% to 60% hemoglobin A, 2% to 3% hemoglobin A_2, 40% to 45% hemoglobin S
    C. 0% hemoglobin A, 0% hemoglobin A_2, 45% to 50% hemoglobin S, 45% to 50% hemoglobin C
    D. 90% to 98% hemoglobin A, 2% to 3% hemoglobin A2, 2% to 3% hemoglobin F

131. The amino acid defect in sickle cell disease is a substitution in the sixth amino acid position of the β-globin chain of:
    A. Leucine for valine
    B. Valine for glycine
    C. Valine for glutamine
    D. Glutamine for valine

132. Which of the following events in the natural course of sickle cell disease significantly increases the risk of infection by encapsulated organisms?
    A. Aplastic anemia
    B. Chronic hemolysis
    C. Chronic penicillin prophylaxis
    D. Splenic autoinfarction

ID/CC: 16-year-old boy presents to urgent care clinic complaining of left knee pain and a limp.

HPI: S.F. was well until about 2 weeks ago when he began to develop intermittent left knee pain mostly while walking. The pain has worsened over the past day and made it uncomfortable to walk. When asked to point to exactly where it hurts, he is vague in pointing to his left knee and says he cannot exactly pinpoint the source. He denies any history of recent trauma or previous injuries to that leg. He also denies any sports-related injuries, especially because he is currently out of sports and working on his "overweight" problem. He has had no fevers or other intercurrent illnesses and is not sexually active.

PMHx:/PSHx: None   **Meds:** None   **All:** NKDA

FHx: No family history of endocrine, rheumatologic, or oncologic disorders.

SHx: Lives at home with mother (divorced) and younger brother, age 10; healthy. Attends 10th grade.

VS: Temp 98.6°F, BP 120/81, HR 77, RR 22

PE: *Gen:* obese adolescent boy sitting in no apparent distress, awake, alert, and oriented × 3. *Ext:* left leg: Limited range of motion with poor abduction, flexion, and internal rotation of hip. Minimal pain on manipulation but tendency toward external rotation of femur as left hip is flexed. Left knee: normal range of motion, no pain on palpation of joint. Normal exam of right leg and normal sensory exam of both legs. Remainder of exam normal.

THOUGHT QUESTIONS

- What is in this patient's differential diagnosis?
- What would be the appropriate radiologic study to obtain at this time? (Consider appropriate views.)
- What is the significance of the perception of knee pain in this patient?

This patient's differential diagnosis includes trauma, slipped capital femoral epiphysis (SCFE), Legg-Calvé-Perthes disease (avascular necrosis of the femoral head), toxic synovitis of the hip. SCFE is a disorder seen early in puberty, whereas Legg-Calvé-Perthes disease generally presents between 4 to 11 years of age.

The appropriate radiologic studies to order are anterior posterior pelvic x-rays in the neutral and frog-leg position to properly view the femoral head.

The pain this patient perceives in his knee is known as "referred" pain. With certain injuries, the patient perceives the pain to occur at a joint other than at the actual site of injury. This misperception is due to convergence of sensory pathways that conduct pain sensation to the CNS. It is therefore important to examine, and image, the entire limb even when only a single joint is reported to hurt. This is especially important to keep in mind when examining children, who are often poor at localizing pain.

CASE CONTINUED

X-ray left hip: AP view—slight widening of epiphyseal physis of femoral head. Frog-leg view—posterior shift of femoral head, displaced 1 cm but less than 2/3 width of femoral neck. Appears as if "an ice cream scoop is falling off the cone." Left knee and left foot—normal.

Based on the x-ray findings, you determine that this patient has a slipped capital femoral epiphysis (SCFE).

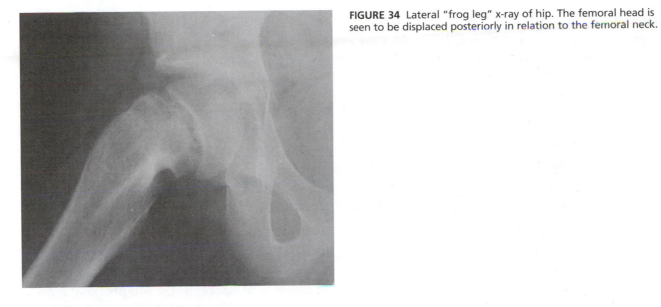

FIGURE 34 Lateral "frog leg" x-ray of hip. The femoral head is seen to be displaced posteriorly in relation to the femoral neck.

QUESTIONS

133. The next course of action would be:
    A. No medications and ask the patient to return for repeat x-rays in 1 week.
    B. Prescribe Motrin and ask patient to return for repeat x-rays in 1 week.
    C. Prescribe Motrin and ask patient to return for orthopedic appointment in 1 week.
    D. Consult an orthopedic surgeon immediately for surgical repair.

134. All of the following characteristics of SCFE are true *except*:
    A. Trauma is a cause of SCFE.
    B. A combination of mechanical and hormonal factors accounts for this lesion.
    C. Males are affected more commonly than females.
    D. Bilateral involvement is common in 15% to 25% of cases.

135. The goal of surgical repair of SCFE is:
    A. Pinning the femoral head in place to prevent further slipping
    B. Pinning of the femoral neck to the femoral shaft to prevent fracture
    C. Re-aligning and pinning of the femoral head
    D. Total joint replacement

136. Which of the following conditions can be a long-term complication of SCFE?
    A. Immune-mediated osteoarthritis of the femoral joint
    B. Avascular necrosis of the femoral head
    C. Loss of pain sensation in affected leg
    D. Loss of proprioception (toe-up, toe-down) in affected foot

ID/CC: 8-year-old girl presents to emergency room at midnight complaining of difficulty walking.

HPI: G.B. was well until 3 weeks ago when she developed a sore throat and fever. She then traveled with her family to Washington, Oregon, Idaho, and Nevada (no camping) and returned 5 days ago with increased tiredness, back pain, neck pain, and irritability. Her mother recalls that G.B. was "list-less" and complained of a vague pain in both legs 3 days ago. When asked where it hurt, she states her legs "just feel tired." Today her mother has had to help support her while walking home from school and walking to the hospital.

PMHx:/PSHx: None   **Meds:** None   **All:** NKDA

FHx: No history of neurologic disorders or CNS malignancies.

SHx: Lives at home with mother, father, and 2 younger brothers, ages 2 and 4, both recovering from viral illness. Attends 3rd grade.

VS: Temp 98.8°F, BP 99/66, HR 80, RR 25

PE: *Gen:* awake, alert, and oriented × 3; lying down, no distress. *Neck:* supple, no nuchal rigidity. *HEENT:* fundi normal, throat slightly erythematous, no exudates. *Ext:* arms (bilateral): normal sensory exam and reflexes; motor strength slightly decreased (4 out of 5) at hands, distal and proximal arms. *Legs* (bilateral): sensory exam: normal exam to pain and light-touch. *Motor exam:* decreased strength in feet, lower, and upper legs (2 out of 5; unable to move against gravity). *Reflex exam:* absent deep tenon reflex (DTR) at Achilles' tendon and patellar tendon. *Proprioceptive exam:* normal "toe-up" and "toe-down" recognition. *Babinski toe reflex:* "downward" direction. *Gait:* unable to walk. Remainder of exam normal.

THOUGHT QUESTIONS

- What is in this patient's differential diagnosis?
- What could be the significance, if any, of whether she had gone camping?
- What are important laboratory tests to consider at this time?

This patient's examination shows symmetric bilateral ascending weakness, with intact sensation and absent reflexes. With this type of exam, her differential diagnosis includes: immune-mediated demyelinating neuropathy (Guillain-Barré syndrome), tick paralysis, spinal cord compression, transverse myelitis, acute cerebellar ataxia, myasthenia gravis, poliomyelitis, botulism, diphtheric neuropathy, and porphyria.

The significance of whether this patient had gone camping may help to direct the differential diagnosis toward tick-borne paralyses.

A CBC with differential, blood culture, and spinal tap for CSF are important laboratory considerations that will help distinguish between the above possibilities.

CASE CONTINUED

Labs: WBC 5400, 64% segs, 17 lymphs, 10 monos, 7 atypical lymphs; plts 270,000. CSF: Gram's stain negative, 1 RBC, 2 WBC, glucose 57, protein 215 g/dL (normal 20–170 g/dL)

You repeat a physical examination and find no evidence of any ticks or tick bites. Given no history of trauma, no signs of upper motor neuron dysfunction, no acute infection, and no RBC abnormalities, you determine this patient must have Guillain-Barré syndrome (the CSF protein levels are usually elevated after the first week of illness).

The patient is admitted to the hospital with increasing lower extremity weakness and gradually worsening upper extremity weakness and areflexia of all limbs. You have chosen to admit her to the pediatric intensive care unit primarily because you are concerned of the possibility that she could develop respiratory failure requiring intubation and mechanical ventilation (12% to 20% of patients).

She remains in the hospital for 3 weeks during which time she was treated with close monitoring, intravenous immunoglobulin (IVIG), and plasmapheresis and is finally discharged and recovers completely normal function by another 2 weeks as an outpatient.

QUESTIONS

137. This patient did *not* have an upper motor neuron lesion because:
    A. Her CSF protein level is 215 g/dL.
    B. She had a "downward" Babinski reflex.
    C. Her DTRs are absent.
    D. Her sensory exam is normal.

138. Although usually of unknown origins, Guillain-Barré syndrome has been associated in 20% to 40% of cases with serologic evidence of recent infection by:
    A. *Streptococcus pneumoniae*
    B. *Staphylococcus aureus*
    C. *Clostridium botulinum*
    D. *Campylobacter jejuni*

139. This patient's recovery of function could have been predicted to occur as:
    A. Progress in the direction of onset (ascending weakness pattern followed by ascending recovery pattern)
    B. Progress in the direction opposite of onset (ascending weakness pattern followed by descending recovery pattern)
    C. Simultaneous recovery of all limbs together
    D. No particular pattern

140. Which of the following autonomic abnormalities is *not* associated with Guillain-Barré syndrome?
    A. Blurry vision
    B. Bowel/bladder dysfunction
    C. Systemic blood pressure changes (hypotension or hypertension)
    D. Abnormal sweating

ID/CC: 17-month-old boy who hasn't started walking.

HPI: P.L. was brought in by his mother over concern that her son was not yet walking. He recently was started in a daycare, where the mother noticed that he was "less advanced than the other children his age." He will cruise briefly on his own, but refuses to walk independently. Over the last several months, she has also noticed him to be more irritable and "colicky." His appetite has decreased over this time period, and his mother has noticed very little weight gain. He had been otherwise healthy, and she hasn't sought medical attention since his 12-month visit.

PMHx: Uncomplicated SVD at term, no chronic illness or hospitalizations.

Meds: None   **All:** NKDA   **Immunizations:** UTD

DietHx: "Loves to put almost anything in his mouth; not lately interested in eating much."

DevHx: Cruising and pulling to stand, not independently walking, only says "mama-dada" specifically and two to three other words, likes to play pat-a-cake, "refuses to play ball. He won't let go and throw it."

FHx: Noncontributory

VS: Temp 98.8°F, BP 90/45, HR 110, RR 28; Weight 9.5 kg (5%)

PE: *Gen:* alert but not very interactive, in no acute distress. *HEENT:* NCAT, nondysmorphic, EOMI, PERRL. *Lungs:* no crackles, no wheeze. *CV:* RR&R, normal S_1, S_2, no murmur. *Abdomen:* soft, nondistended/nontender, normal active bowel sounds (NABS), no masses or visceromegaly. *Skin:* no bruises or lesions noted, no clubbing, cyanosis, or edema. *Neuro:* normal tone/strength/reflexes, somewhat unsteady truncal posture, responsive to voice but not to commands. *ROS:* occasional vomiting "due likely to feeding him new foods," no diarrhea, occasional bouts of constipation.

THOUGHT QUESTIONS

- What further components of the history or physical examination would you pursue?
- What is in your differential diagnosis at this point?
- What diagnostic evaluations may aid you in your diagnosis?

For a patient who is suspected of not meeting developmental milestones, the history should include a thorough review of the presenting complaint and a review of systems. In addition, a family history of other children or members with any developmentally related problems should be obtained. A social and environmental history should note the child's caretakers, stressors, and learning/playing/living environs. It is also important to note perceptions of hearing and vision. The thorough physical examination should particularly focus on neurologic findings, growth, and developmental maturity. The differential diagnosis in children with global developmental delays is wide, but mainly includes cerebral dysgenesis, hypoxic-ischemic encephalopathy, chromosomal anomalies, metabolic derangements, congenital infections, and toxin exposures. Evaluations that may be useful are a thorough developmental examination, CT or MRI, and directed laboratory tests (such as CBC, metabolic tests, chromosome analysis, toxin levels).

CASE CONTINUED

A developmental examination revealed: positive protective reflexes, clumsy pincer grasp, would not build tower of cubes or mark/imitate with crayons, no imitative behavior, and did not know any body parts. A CT scan was performed that was normal. Further environmental history revealed that the family had moved to a new home 5 months ago, which was undergoing partial renovation and restoration. The home had been built in 1928. Suspecting exposure to lead-based paint/dust, a serum lead test was done. A level of 90 was found, and the child was diagnosed lead poisoning.

Developmental delay is defined as performance significantly below average in a given skill area. These skill areas are divided into four domains: gross motor, fine/visual motor, language, and social. Although there may be numerous causes for global developmental delay, a significant number of cases may have no cause, particularly for those patients with delay in isolated domains. It is important to note critical ages and the expected milestones associated with them. This patient had global developmental delay for his age.

QUESTIONS

141. Which of the following is least likely to be associated with lead poisoning?
    A. Macrocytic anemia
    B. Decreased cognitive ability
    C. Decreased coordination
    D. GI symptoms
    E. Pica

142. Which of the following is the best indicator for future intellectual achievement?
    A. Fine motor development
    B. Gross motor development
    C. Language development
    D. Social development

143. Which of the following statements regarding cerebral palsy are *false*?
    A. Always involves motor areas of the brain
    B. Always is associated with mental retardation
    C. 20% to 30% of cases are idiopathic
    D. Motor problems are static rather than progressive
    E. Requires multidisciplinary approach to therapy

144. List the proper sequence for sexual development in males:
    A. Development of pubic hair
    B. Penile enlargement
    C. Testicular enlargement
    D. Height growth spurt

ID/CC: 6-year-old boy is brought in by his parents for limping for a week, and now with "dark urine."

HPI: G.N. has been limping and complaining of a blister on his left heel for a week, but was otherwise in good health until yesterday when he began to feel tired and his mother thought he looked "puffy." He has been drinking well, but has only urinated a very small amount of brownish urine once today. G.N. complains of a mild headache, but has not had fever, rash, abdominal pain, joint pain, dysuria, diarrhea, or vomiting. There is no history of trauma, and he has never had dark urine before. His parents are concerned that the blister has not healed and now appears infected.

PMHx: No illnesses or hospitalizations.

Meds: None   **All:** NKDA   **Immunizations:** UTD

VS: Temp 36.8°C (98.2°F), BP 130/80 (90–115/65–70), HR 90, RR 22; Weight 22 kg (65%)

PE: *Gen:* a tired-appearing but nontoxic boy. *HEENT:* mild periorbital edema. Oropharynx is moist, without erythema or exudate, no lymphadenopathy. *CV:* RR&R without murmur, pulses and cap refill brisk. *Lungs:* clear. *Abdomen:* no abdominal or flank tenderness or bruising. No organomegaly. *Ext:* no dependent edema, joint and muscle exam are normal. A small superficial honey-crusted erosion is visible on the left heel; it is mildly tender, with 1 cm of surrounding erythema. Remainder of exam is within normal limits.

THOUGHT QUESTIONS

- What system seems to be predominantly affected in this child?
- What is your differential diagnosis and how will you further evaluate him?

G.N.'s symptoms—dark urine, reduced urine output (oliguria), edema, and hypertension—suggest renal pathology. Dark urine usually signifies hematuria, which has a broad differential. Causes of hematuria in children include infection, trauma, stones, hematologic disorders, benign or familial hematuria, and menses. In this case, the lack of pain, fever, or significant medical history, and the presence of additional symptoms suggesting a decrease in glomerular function (i.e., edema, oliguria, and hypertension) should raise concern for either nephrotic syndrome or glomerulonephritis.

Nephrotic syndrome, a noninflammatory and usually idiopathic condition, is characterized by massive proteinuria and hypoalbuminemia. Periorbital swelling and eventually generalized edema are usually the presenting complaints; hypertension and hematuria are less common. Glomerulonephritis (GN), which refers to inflammation of the glomerular basement membrane (GBM), is usually immune-complex mediated. Hematuria is the hallmark of this disease, and proteinuria may be present but is much less severe than in nephrotic syndrome. The urine itself is a valuable tool in differentiating nephrotic syndrome from GN. Additional labs should be directed toward evaluating the patient's electrolyte and fluid status, and further characterization of the source of his renal disease.

CASE CONTINUED

You ascertain from the boy's mother that there is no family history of rheumatologic disease, renal disease, diabetes, or deafness. Meanwhile, you send the urine sample to the laboratory for urinalysis and culture. The urinalysis shows numerous red blood cell casts, a few white cell casts, no bacteria, and small protein. You also draw a CBC, electrolytes, and an albumin level, which are all within normal limits except for slightly elevated BUN and creatinine of 25 and 1.0, respectively. Based on these results, you suspect glomerulonephritis (GN) and send a C3 complement level, which comes back low, confirming the presence of inflammation with consumption of complement.

THOUGHT QUESTION

- What is the most likely cause of this patient's glomerulonephritis?

The most common cause of acute GN in children is poststreptococcal glomerulonephritis (PSGN). Other less common causes of GN in children include IgA nephropathy, lupus, and Alport syndrome (a hereditary progressive form of the disease often accompanied by deafness). This patient's clinical picture and history of a recent skin infection support the diagnosis of PSGN. His laboratory results are consistent with this diagnosis as well, with red cell casts and a depressed C3 level. You send an ASO (antistreptolysin O) titer, which confirms the diagnosis. G.N. is then started on antibiotics and begun on outpatient management for his renal disease.

QUESTIONS

145. Management of PSGN
    A. Rarely prevents renal failure
    B. Should include steroids
    C. Involves aggressive fluid rehydration
    D. Is mainly supportive

146. Signs of acute renal failure include each of the following *except*:
    A. Azotemia (elevated BUN and creatinine)
    B. Hyperkalemia
    C. Increased urine output
    D. Edema

147. The most common cause of nephrotic syndrome in children is
    A. Minimal change disease
    B. Membranous GN
    C. NSAIDs
    D. Lupus

148. Complications of nephrotic syndrome include
    A. Bacterial infections
    B. Thrombosis
    C. End-stage renal disease
    D. All of the above

ID/CC: 15-month-old girl has been refusing to walk for the last 4 days.

HPI: O.M. is a previously active child who seems well and happy when she is sitting or lying down, but will not walk to her parents or to get toys, and she cries when placed on her feet. She has also had a low-grade fever for a week, which her parents were told was due to a viral infection. O.M. has had a good appetite, but recently has seemed more tired. She has not had runny nose, cough, rash, joint swelling, vomiting, or diarrhea. The parents say they have not seen her fall, although she is such an active child that she often gets away from them.

PMHx: No hospitalizations or surgeries   **Meds:** Tylenol for fever

All: NKDA   **Immunizations:** UTD   **SHx:** Noncontributory

---

THOUGHT QUESTION

- What will you look for on physical examination?

In this toddler who seems to be refusing to walk due to pain, the source of her discomfort may be anywhere from the lumbar spine to the bottom of the feet. The physical examination should include a careful assessment of this region to characterize any tenderness, weakness, swelling or deformity in the lower extremities. Observation is a crucial part of this examination; note the child's position of comfort, and any spontaneous use of the limbs. The remainder of the examination should assess the child's general health and stability, as well as look for stigmata of systemic disease or trauma such as rash, bruising, organomegaly, and lymphadenopathy.

VS: Temp 38.8°C (101.8°F) HR 120, RR 25; Weight 11 kg (75%)

PE: *Gen:* a playful, healthy appearing child, who cries when pulled to a stand and holds her right leg off the ground. *HEENT:* no lymphadenopathy, normocephalic, oropharynx normal. *CV:* RR&R, no murmur. *Lungs:* clear. *Skin:* warm and pink, no bruising or rashes. *Ext:* no redness, swelling warmth, or limitation in movement of the lower extremity joints. The spine is palpated without discomfort. There is no redness, swelling, or deformity of the legs or feet. Careful examination of the lower right leg reveals pain on palpation of the proximal tibia.

THOUGHT QUESTIONS

- What is your differential diagnosis at this point?
- What further studies would you obtain?

Based on your exam and the history, you are particularly concerned about a process in the bone of the lower leg. Possibilities include infection (e.g., osteomyelitis, septic arthritis), malignancy (e.g., leukemia, metastatic neuroblastoma), or trauma. A plain film of the leg is a good diagnostic test to start with. It may reveal fracture, a lytic lesion in the bone, or some of the early signs of bone infection such as periosteal reaction and tissue plane elevation. More sophisticated imaging such as nuclear bone scan or MRI may be indicated to identify subtle bony changes, or to further distinguish between infectious and destructive processes. A CBC, blood culture, and ESR should be performed to evaluate for infection, inflammation, and possible bone marrow involvement.

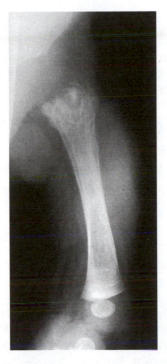

FIGURE 38 X-ray of femur showing periosteal elevation. Used with permission from Rudolf M, Levene M. Paediatrics and Child Health. Oxford: Blackwell Science, Ltd., 1999: 223.

CASE CONTINUED

The CBC shows an elevated WBC count of 18K, with 87% neutrophils. The ESR is elevated at 102. A plain film of the right leg shows elevation of soft tissue planes around the tibial metaphysis, indicating an inflammatory process in the bone. Due to concern for osteomyelitis, an orthopedic consult is obtained and the child is taken to the operating room for needle aspiration of the bone, which recovers *S. aureus*. The child is admitted to the hospital for parenteral therapy with nafcillin. The blood culture subsequently grows *S. aureus*. After 1 week of parenteral therapy, with good response, the patient is discharged home on oral antibiotics to complete 14 to 21 days of therapy.

QUESTIONS

149. Most cases of osteomyelitis in children
    A. Occur in children >5 years of age
    B. Are viral in origin
    C. Are hematogenous in origin
    D. Involve the flat bones

150. Risk factors for osteomyelitis include each of the following *except*:
    A. Female sex
    B. Recent trauma to the bone
    C. Impaired host defenses
    D. Previous orthopedic surgery

151. Possible consequences of osteomyelitis include:
    A. Impaired bone growth
    B. Chronic or recurrent infection
    C. Pathologic fracture
    D. All of the above

152. Osteomyelitis in the neonate
    A. Is usually caused by group B *Streptococcus*
    B. Is usually accompanied by fever
    C. Often involves more than one bone
    D. Is easy to diagnose

ID/CC: 22-month-old baby boy brought to emergency room at 3 AM by parents following 5 minutes of generalized seizure.

HPI: Parents state that their toddler, F.S., was well until last evening when they noted a runny nose, watery eyes, and slightly increased irritability with refusal to eat dinner. At 2:30 AM they heard him cry and then suddenly become silent. When they reached his room they found that his eyes were rolled back, and he had rhythmic jerking of both his arms and legs lasting at least 5 minutes. He did not stop breathing but turned slightly pale. Before they could dial 911 the episode stopped, so they rushed him into the emergency room, where he continued to intermittently cry and sleep. When asked if he had a fever, the mother said that he did feel warm to the touch. He had been otherwise healthy with no coughing, vomiting, diarrhea, or rashes and has not had any known ill contacts.

PMHx: Birth history unremarkable: full term, SVD Apgar 9^1 and 9^5; D/C home on DOL 2.

PSHx: None   **Meds:** None   **All:** NKDA   **Immunizations:** UTD

FHx: No family history of seizures or metabolic disorders.

SHx: Lives at home with healthy mother and father, no siblings. Attends daycare during week.

VS: Temp 102.1°F, BP 90/60, HR 105, RR 40

PE: *Gen:* sleeping quietly, no apparent distress. Awakes easily by briefly opening eyes when addressed loudly. *HEENT:* normocephalic, no bumps, bruises. Eyes watery, no crusting, PERRLA, fundi normal. Clear rhinorrhea from nose. *Neck:* supple. *Lungs:* CTAB. *Abdomen:* soft, nondistended/ nontender, no masses. *Neuro:* normal motor, sensory, and reflex exam. *Ext:* gait, too sleepy to assess.

THOUGHT QUESTIONS

- What is in this patient's differential diagnosis?
- What is the significance of the absence of a postictal state in this patient?

The differential diagnosis of seizures in an infant includes two broad categories: febrile and non-febrile. The term "febrile seizure" refers to a seizure that occurs as a result of a high or rapidly rising fever. Possible causes may therefore include any condition that causes a fever, but do not include certain infectious or noninfectious illnesses (meningitis, encephalitis, toxic encephalopathy) that can also cause fever but cause seizures because of underlying CNS effects. Nonfebrile seizures include these causes, as well as any condition that causes a seizure without fever, such as metabolic derangements, cerebrovascular events, oncologic masses, trauma, or idiopathic epilepsy. Most febrile seizures as well as petit mal (absence seizures) are *not* associated with a postictal state.

CASE CONTINUED

Given the history and presence of a fever, you are aware that the causes with the highest risks for this child's convulsions are meningitis or another CNS infection. Because you elicit no meningeal or encephalopathic signs on examination, and the child is not ill-appearing and has now returned to his neurologic baseline, you determine that he has had a febrile seizure. The history and physical findings are consistent with a nonspecific viral syndrome and no further workup is necessary.

THOUGHT QUESTION

- What is the most appropriate management step at this time?

The most important intervention at this time is to provide parental education about febrile seizures. The fever should be controlled with around the clock antipyretics such as acetaminophen (Tylenol) or ibuprofen for the duration of the viral illness to prevent further seizures. Aspirin should be avoided secondary to a risk of developing Reye syndrome. Children with simple febrile seizures require no further evaluation beyond determination of the source of the fever. Complicated febrile seizures, however, should have additional workup (including lumbar puncture) and close follow-up, because there is more likely to be an underlying condition that makes the child more vulnerable to seizures.

QUESTIONS

153. All of the following are true regarding febrile seizures *except*:
    A. Febrile seizures occur in 2% to 4% of young children in developed countries.
    B. Febrile seizures are always classified as simple, nonfocal seizures.
    C. After the first febrile seizure, about one-third of children will experience one or more recurrences.
    D. Most recurrences (75%) of febrile seizure occur within a year.

154. Febrile seizures most commonly occur in children aged:
    A. Birth through 1 month
    B. 1 month through 6 months
    C. 6 months through 5 years
    D. 5 years through 10 years

155. An EEG obtained from a child who has just had a febrile seizure will most likely be:
    A. Normal
    B. Showing a characteristic three-spikes-per-second waveform
    C. Showing generalized slowing
    D. Showing generalized slowing with occasional sharp waves

156. During the early months of life, the excitability of the newborn cortex:
    A. Decreases gradually
    B. Increases continually into and beyond adulthood
    C. Increases initially and then decreases in the second decade of life
    D. Does not change

ID/CC: 1-month-old baby boy presents to emergency room at midnight appearing pale and gray.

HPI: V.M., a full-term infant born 1 month ago, was in his usual state of good health until about 24 hours ago when his mother reports that he began to feed poorly. He normally breastfeeds about 20 minutes per breast at least every 4 to 6 hours, but over the past 24 hours he has refused to feed for more than 5 minutes per breast, no more than only every 8 hours. She does not report any fevers, and in fact, the baby's father has just recovered from a cold during the past week. She has also noted that he is not urinating, with the last wet diaper nearly 18 hours ago. He normally has a wet diaper at least every 2 to 3 hours. This evening, he became increasingly more fussy and refused to feed altogether. Within a couple of hours his color became pale and gray, and he was unresponsive. The parents called 911, and a paramedics team intubated him, started an IV, and rushed him to the hospital emergency room. He had no vomiting or diarrhea, no obvious signs of any blood loss, and no history of trauma or toxic ingestions. He had a normal delivery following an uncomplicated pregnancy with good prenatal care.

PMHx:/PSHx: None   **Meds:** None   **All:** NKDA

FHx: No family history of congenital heart diseases or metabolic diseases.

SHx: Lives at home with mother and father, no siblings. At home with mother during day.

THOUGHT QUESTIONS

- What is in this patient's differential diagnosis?
- What are the three fundamental steps during a proper resuscitation?

This patient's differential diagnosis includes conditions that present as shock. Shock is classified into four major categories: hypovolemic, cardiogenic, distributive, and septic. Hypovolemic shock occurs from water and electrolyte losses such as vomiting and diarrhea or hemorrhage. Cardiogenic shock results from congenital heart diseases, ischemic heart diseases with cardiomyopathies, or arrhythmias. Distributive shock occurs from anaphylaxis, neurologic injury, or drug toxicity. Septic shock results from the common pathogens that cause infection within particular age groups.

The first three steps during any resuscitative procedure are A, B, and C: Airway, Breathing, and Circulation. Performed in this order, these should be the necessary steps in initiating any resuscitation. Establishing an airway in an obtunded individual usually requires intubation via endotracheal tube. Breathing refers to actually ensuring that once an airway is established, the patient is able to either breathe spontaneously, or breathe with the assistance of mechanical ventilation. Circulation involves the assessment of the adequacy of proper perfusion to the vital organs and establishing IV access, or rarely, intraosseus access to deliver fluids and medication.

VS: Temp 97°F, BP 50/30, HR 180, RR 70

PE: *Gen:* sleepy, unresponsive to gentle touch, withdraws appropriately to pain. *HEENT:* intubated, mucous membranes dry, eyes mildly sunken, throat nonerythematous. *Lungs:* crackles at bases bilaterally; good air entry. *CV:* tachycardia, RR&R, normal S_1, S_2, ventricular S_3 gallop. No murmur. *Abdomen:* soft, nondistended, minimal bowel sounds, no masses. Liver edge down 4 to 5 cm below costal margin. No palpable spleen tip. *Skin:* sweaty, cool extremities, capillary refill time 5 to 6 sec.

THOUGHT QUESTION
- What is the significance of the sweating, ventricular S₃ gallop, and the low liver edge?

Taken together, this constellation of clinical findings suggests a patient with congestive heart failure. It would be helpful to obtain a chest x-ray, electrocardiogram (ECG), and an echocardiogram to detect pulmonary edema, measure relative forces, and assess heart function.

CASE CONTINUED

Labs: *Chest x-ray:* pulmonary edema, enlarged heart size. *ECG:* ST segment depression, T wave inversion. *Echocardiogram:* decreased contractility of left ventricle and moderately decreased ejection fraction.

After no improvement in condition despite adequate volume resuscitation, a normal CBC and negative blood culture, you determine this patient has congestive heart failure and shock due to the cardiogenic cause of myocarditis. The patient was probably exposed to the same viral infection that had affected her father earlier. ST segment depression indicates that the heart has sustained ischemic changes.

QUESTIONS

157. The most common cause of myocarditis in North American children is due to:
    A. Adenovirus
    B. Coxsackie A virus
    C. Coxsackie B virus
    D. Respiratory syncytial virus
    E. Rhinovirus

158. Which of the following vascular beds is *not* considered a vital end organ?
    A. Hepatic
    B. Coronary
    C. Cerebral
    D. Renal

159. The level of which of the following is the most sensitive measure of intravascular fluid status?
    A. Tachypnea
    B. Tachycardia
    C. Urine output
    D. Consciousness

160. Which of the following is *not* considered a resuscitation medication for septic shock?
    A. Glucose infusion
    B. Antibiotics
    C. Normal saline
    D. Lactated Ringer's solution

ID/CC: 14-month-old girl with 1-day history of irritability.

HPI: C.A. was brought in to the emergency department by her mother after she was noted this morning to be increasingly irritable. She refuses to eat or drink, and when not crying, "she is very tired, and not interacting with me as much as she normally does." She had been cruising (walking) for the last 2 to 3 weeks, but now cries when she is left to stand. She has had no fever and no other symptoms of illness. The mother was concerned about the irritability and her inability to console the infant. She tried giving the baby acetaminophen this morning, without any relief. She has brought her in for visits in the past regarding irritability, and a "strange rash on her back and legs." A careful review of systems reveals no other symptoms. The mother reveals that her husband, from whom she is separated, took care of the child this past weekend till this morning. He usually takes care of the infant every weekend. By phone, he describes her as being playful this past weekend, but that she "may have climbed onto the sofa and fallen down this morning." He does not know of any rashes.

PMHx: Born at 28 weeks' GA, neonate intensive care unit stay for 2 months

Meds: Albuterol as needed, inhaled corticosteroids, acetaminophen as above

All: NKDA   **Immunizations:** UTD, received RSV prophylaxis last winter

DevHx: Global mild developmental delay (babble/coos, starting to cruise).

VS: Temp 98.8°F, BP 115/60, HR 150, RR 30

PE: *Gen:* alert, but uncomfortable; crying and difficult to examine; appears small for age. *HEENT:* NCAT, EOMI, tympanic membranes within normal limits, oropharynx clear. *Skin/Ext:* refuses to move right leg or bear weight, cries upon palpation of right middle thigh, which appears swollen; multiple linear (1 cm) paired scars on buttocks and lower extremities of varying age, circular bluish discolorations on back.

THOUGHT QUESTIONS

- What currently lies in your differential diagnosis?
- What laboratory studies/evaluations and treatment is indicated for this child?

Changes in behavior warrant suspicion of any infectious causes, including meningoencephalitis. Also, seizure activity and CNS disturbances, trauma, ingestions/toxic exposures, GI disturbances (such as intussusception), and metabolic disturbances should be included. In this case, nonaccidental trauma should be strongly suspected in this child, as the clinical examination and history do not match appropriately. To evaluate this possibility, a detailed physical examination and skeletal survey (generally x-rays of the long bones, skull, spine, thorax, pelvis, and extremities) should be performed.

CASE CONTINUED

The skeletal survey reveals a spiral fracture of the right humerus and multiple old symmetric fractures of the posterior ribs. On closer examination, the infant's "rash" is suspiciously consistent with burn marks from contact with a cigarette lighter. You are further suspicious when you recall that the child is developmentally incapable of climbing onto an elevated surface and that fractures occurring before true ambulation are usually inflicted. You conclude that this child has been subjected to nonaccidental trauma and notify Child Protective Services. The infant is admitted to the hospital for further management, which includes a CT scan of the head and ophthalmologic exam (for suspicion of sequelae of shaken baby syndrome).

> **THOUGHT QUESTIONS**
> * What are the risk factors for nonaccidental trauma?
> * What is your legal responsibility as a physician?

Nonaccidental trauma and physical abuse is an unfortunate cause of mortality and morbidity. Almost half of children brought for medical attention as a result of physical abuse are under age 1. Parents, male paramours, and step-parents are the most common perpetrators. Other types of abuse include sexual abuse, emotional abuse, and neglect (which actually results in more deaths than sexual and physical abuse combined). Risk factors include chronic disease/prematurity, age younger than 3 years, perception of the child as "difficult" or "abnormal," single parents, and history of abuse in the parent or caregiver.

Incompatibility of history with injury or clinical examination and delay in seeking attention warrant suspicion of abuse. Physical findings of burns and other injuries (bruises, lacerations) in specific patterns (imprints of a stricken object) or locations (lesions on low-trauma areas such as the buttocks or back) suggest abuse. A thorough examination and workup for sexual abuse should include evaluation for sexually transmitted diseases (STDs). Radiographic findings of spiral and metaphyseal chip fractures are virtually diagnostic of abuse. Rib and skull fractures can result from abuse as well. Healthcare workers are legally required to report any suspicion of abuse or neglect to the appropriate child protective agencies, and this should be the first course of action. Often children are immediately placed in a hospital for protective custody until a safe environment can be established.

QUESTIONS

161. Which of the following conditions can be confused with nonaccidental trauma?
    A. Osteogenesis imperfecta
    B. Coagulopathies
    C. Mongolian spots
    D. Folk remedies causing bruising
    E. All of the above

162. Which of the following is a risk factor for a child to be abused?
    A. Age <3 years old
    B. Chronic illness or disease
    C. Foster children
    D. Low socioeconomic status
    E. All of the above

163. Which of the following is consistent with findings of shaken baby syndrome?
    A. Subdural hematomas
    B. Metaphyseal chip fractures
    C. Retinal hemorrhages
    D. Usually little or no evidence of external injury
    E. All of the above

164. Which of the following statements is *true*?
    A. Failure to thrive and developmental delay can result from child abuse.
    B. Nonaccidental burns are usually superficial and in a splash and droplet pattern.
    C. Common bruises from childhood play usually are not on bony-protuberances.
    D. Crying and toilet training are uncommon triggers for abuse.

ID/CC: 14-year-old boy with confusion and vomiting.

HPI: E.H. is brought in by his parents and a friend for increasing confusion and episode of vomiting after a skateboarding accident in which he fell and hit his head. He was not wearing a helmet at the time, remembers falling backward of a staircase railing and hitting the left side of his head. A friend claims that he was briefly unconscious, but awoke seconds later. In the hour following the accident, he has been more "confused" according to his parents, he has vomited once, and complains of a "major headache."

PMHx: History of asthma and eczema.　**Meds:** None　**All:** None

FHx: Maternal grandfather with stroke. Paternal grandmother with Alzheimer disease.

THOUGHT QUESTIONS

- What further history would you elicit at this point?
- What is your differential diagnosis?

The history given by the parents and patient in this case seem consistent, but ideally the source of injury should be described by the child and caretaker separately (inconsistencies should raise suspicions of abuse). An accurate account of the mechanism of injury and the immediate events following are important. Loss of consciousness should be elucidated, as well as amnesia, seizures, and visual impairment. Any changes in mental status (including confusion, inappropriate words, and changes in orientation) should be noted. Vomiting, headache, and changes in mental status suggest increased intracranial pressure. As with any painful symptom, the specific components of the headache should be further described.

The differential diagnosis for confused states and vomiting should include trauma and abuse, causes of encephalopathy and encephalitis, meningitis, toxic ingestion, and vascular anomalies leading to hemorrhage. Intracranial masses should be associated with insidious progress of symptoms. In most cases, a thorough history will narrow this list to the appropriate diagnosis and course of action. Evaluation of the child with suspected head trauma starts with the ABCs (airway, breathing, circulation), and brief but thorough history, and subsequent physical examination and secondary survey.

CASE CONTINUED

Upon further questioning, the patient and parents deny any seizure activity, claim that the headache is mostly concentrated at the site of the injury. His family has no history of epilepsy or neurologic problems. He has been otherwise well and without any complaints, except some pain at his left wrist. He denies any toxic exposures or habits.

VS: Temp 99°F, BP 110/70, HR 80, RR 24

PE: *Gen:* supine, sleepy but responsive, alert and oriented to name and place. *HEENT:* laceration behind left ear lobe, tenderness on occiput and left mastoid, with posterior auricular bruising on left side. No CSF rhinorrhea or otorrhea. PERRL/EOMI. *Neck:* supple, full range of motion. *Abdomen:* soft, nondistended/nontender, no visceromegaly, positive bowel sounds. *Back:* spine straight, no bruises. *Skin/Ext:* palpable pain at left wrist, decreased ability to extend wrist, anatomical snuffbox tenderness. *Neuro:* CN 2–12 grossly intact. He has mild bilateral lateral visual field deficits; deep tenon reflex and strength response are normal; he seems confused as to what time of day it is, and asks "whether or not you've seen my chicken." He becomes more combative during your exam and cannot recall his parents' names nor can he do any complex functions (serial 7s). His gait is unsteady and he seems to veer left.

THOUGHT QUESTION
- What further laboratory studies/evaluations and treatment would you perform on this patient at this point?

This patient, mainly due to his confusion and clinical exam, has a CT scan of his head and C-spine which reveals a left basilar skull fracture and an epidural hematoma. Neurosurgical assistance is sought immediately. Incidentally, he also suffered a left navicular bone fracture in his wrist, further highlighting the importance of a full body examination and secondary survey.

A concussion is defined as a brief loss of consciousness after head injury associated with antero-grade or retrograde amnesia. Brain injury is not detectable, in contrast to cerebral contusions. Hemorrhage occurring after trauma is usually epidural or subdural rather than intraparenchymal. Physical signs and clinical evidence can suggest the diagnosis, but a CT scan of the head is the imaging choice for an expeditious therapeutic course. Intracranial pressure (ICP) reduction and monitoring may often be required for the patient with cerebral edema. The child with a history of loss of consciousness or abnormal neurologic findings should be observed in the hospital setting.

QUESTIONS

165. The primary determinant of neurologic outcome in head trauma correlates most with:
    A. Size of the hematoma
    B. Associated seizure activity
    C. Length of associated unconsciousness
    D. Mechanical force of the injury

166. Which of the following statements regarding evaluation of head trauma are *false*?
    A. Cranial nerve function may help to localize the injury.
    B. Vomiting, headache, and mental status changes strongly suggest increased ICP.
    C. Cerebral edema is the most important acute complication.
    D. Cervical collar application is usually unnecessary.

167. Which of the following is characteristic of a *subdural* bleed?
    A. Appears as biconcave lesion on CT scan
    B. Associated with rupture of middle meningeal artery
    C. Hematoma occurring between the dura and arachnoid layers
    D. Can be classically with a "lucid interval"

168. Which of the following statements regarding head trauma are *true*?
    A. Cushing's triad is the hallmark of decreased ICP.
    B. Posterior auricular bruising can be a sign suggestive of a cervical spine fracture.
    C. Oxygen, fluid restriction, and head of bed elevation can help reduce ICP.
    D. Hyperventilation and mannitol help to increase ICP.

ID/CC: 12-year-old girl with erratic behavior.

HPI: T.I. is brought into the emergency department by her mother this evening after erratic behavior over the last 2 to 3 days. Her mother states that she has been intermittently tearful, angry, and occasionally confused, muttering to herself repeatedly. Yesterday, she had vomiting (nonbloody and nonbilious), malaise, and no appetite, which all seem to have improved somewhat. There has been no fever, no diarrhea, no ill contacts, and no recent travel, no new foods. Her mother says that she has been silent all evening and becomes excessively angry when approached.

PMHx: Noncontributory   **PSHx:** None   **Meds:** None   **All:** NKDA

VS: Temp 98.8°F, BP 110/65, HR 90, RR 22

PE: *Gen:* quiet, reluctant, but alert and oriented × 3. *HEENT:* NCAT, EOMI, PERRL *Neck:* supple. *Lungs:* normal exam. *CV:* normal exam. *Abdomen:* soft, right upper quadrant and epigastric tenderness with liver edge palpable 3 cm below costal margin, positive bowel sounds, no other masses. *Rectal:* exam normal. *Back/Ext:* mild back pain, otherwise normal. ROS: no dysuria, no headache, no weight loss.

THOUGHT QUESTIONS

- What is in your differential diagnosis?
- What elements of the history are helpful toward making a diagnosis?
- What diagnostic tests may aid in your diagnosis?

The differential diagnosis for this patient would include food poisoning, gastroenteritis, gallstone disease, hepatitis, Epstein-Barr infection, gastritis and peptic ulcer disease, and toxic ingestions. For the patient with erratic behavior or with altered mental status, a thorough history should include an attempt to identify any substance ingested and the specific nature of the ingestion (when? how much? types of substances?) and the subsequent behaviors. This can often be a challenge in the unwitnessed event for a toddler, or in the case of an adolescent. It is helpful to obtain a detailed social history, which including details of the home environment, school, stressors/sexual activity, and toxic exposures as well as history of any trauma. In the patient with altered mental status or behavioral changes, initial screening evaluation may include an accucheck, pulse oximetry, ECG, serum electrolytes and osmolarity, and determination of serum pH. Toxicology screens can also be helpful. In patients like above, other directed laboratory tests that may be helpful are a CBC, urine pregnancy test, urinalysis, liver function tests, and pancreatic enzyme tests.

CASE CONTINUED

Upon further questioning, her mother says her menarche was nearly 2 years ago and she has normal cycles. In the emergency department, you order a CBC and urinalysis which are normal, and a pregnancy test which is negative. Her liver enzymes are greatly elevated (ALT 2100), and her prothrombin time (PT) is mildly elevated at 13.9. A urine toxicology screen for opiates, amphetamines, LSD, and marijuana is negative. Serum levels for aspirin and acetaminophen are undetected. A CT scan of the abdomen is done and is normal. She is still quite angry and tearful and now becomes combative. As you try and calm her down, she reveals that she is scared for herself for "what she did" but that her mother "deserves it!" Further questioning reveals that her parents have decided to file for divorce and the patient subsequently admits to ingesting 15 extra-strength acetaminophen tablets nearly 2.5 days ago. She is admitted, treated, and evaluated by psychiatry for follow-up.

Acute ingestions are challenging, but should be suspected in any patient with altered mental status, acute behavioral changes, seizures, arrhythmias, and coma. Most cases occur in children under 5. Adolescents account for many cases, mostly intentional and often representing a suicide gesture or attempt. It is important to note that multiple substances may be involved. Acetaminophen is a commonly ingested substance, and generally affects the liver via toxic byproducts during metabolism via the cytochrome P450 system, resulting in necrosis and damage. It initially clinically manifests with vomiting/nausea, anorexia, and pallor. This may progress over days to abdominal pain, back pain, and subsequently to signs and symptoms of liver dysfunction. Acetaminophen levels in plasma, particularly noted within 24 hours of a known single-dose ingestion, can be used to extrapolate hepatic toxicity. In many cases, levels may be undetected due to the length of time elapsed since the ingestion. In most cases, with the appropriate treatment, prognosis is excellent.

QUESTIONS

169. The differential diagnosis for acute mental status change usually includes all *except*:
    A. Intracranial hemorrhage
    B. Hypoglycemia
    C. Erythema toxicum neonatorum
    D. Panic disorder
    E. LSD ingestion

170. Which substance is *not* properly matched with its antidote?
    A. Acetaminophen: *N*-acetylcysteine
    B. Opiates: naloxone
    C. Iron: deferoxamine
    D. Diazepam: physostigmine

171. Initial management of acute poisonings may include all of the following *except*:
    A. Assessment of ABCs
    B. EEG
    C. Gastric lavage
    D. Activated charcoal
    E. Induction of emesis

172. Which of the following statements is *true*?
    A. Aspirated hydrocarbons pose little threat to lung tissue.
    B. Home safety rarely prevents ingestions.
    C. Mydriasis, tachycardia, and elevated blood pressure are found in sympathomimetic ingestion.
    D. Activated charcoal can be used for alcohol ingestions.
    E. Mydriasis, tachycardia, and elevated BP are found in cholinergic ingestion.

ID/CC: A.N. is a 15-year-old girl brought in by her mother for "looking thin."

HPI: The girl says everything's fine, and she feels great, but her mother thinks she is wasting away. "A few months ago she was a beautiful girl, now look at her," she says. Mother reports that the patient hardly eats anything any more and seems withdrawn. The patient angrily says she just isn't hungry for dinner when she gets home from track practice, and mother's cooking is "unhealthy." She denies fevers, abdominal pain, diarrhea, vomiting, or headache, but has been mildly constipated. She weighed 110 lbs (50 kg) at her last doctor's visit 9 months ago.

PMHx: No hospitalizations or surgeries.   **Meds:** None   **All:** NKDA

Immunizations: UTD for age

SHx: Sophomore in high school, straight-A student. Runs cross-country for the track team. Parents are lawyers, recently divorced, 10-year-old brother is healthy, but having trouble in school.

VS: Temp 36.0°C (96.8°F), BP 105/70, HR 52 (60–80), RR 14; Weight 42.5 kg (7%), Height 165 cm (60%)

PE: *Gen:* a polite, cooperative, and very thin young lady wearing baggy sweats. *HEENT:* no lymphadenopathy, oropharynx normal. *CV:* bradycardia, regular rhythm, no murmurs. *Lungs:* clear. *Abdomen:* soft with normal bowel sounds, no masses. *Skin:* cool and dry, no rashes or bruising. *GU:* Tanner 5 female, normal external genitalia.

THOUGHT QUESTIONS

- What types of illnesses are you concerned about in this patient?
- What further history would you like to obtain?

Causes of weight loss in teenagers can be considered in two broad categories: organic and nonorganic causes. Organic causes include chronic infection (e.g., TB, HIV, EBV), malignancy (e.g., leukemia, lymphoma, CNS, and bone tumors) endocrine disturbance (e.g., hyperthyroidism, diabetes mellitus, adrenal or pituitary insufficiency) and GI disease (e.g., inflammatory bowel disease, malabsorption). Nonorganic causes include drug use, depression, and eating disorders such as anorexia nervosa and bulimia nervosa.

Because the patient's history and physical examination do not suggest an organic cause, she should be interviewed confidentially without the parent present to obtain an accurate history of dieting behavior, sexual activity, drug use, and any social stressors that may be contributing to emotional disturbance.

CASE CONTINUED

You ask mother to step out of the room and ask A.N. what she thinks is the reason for her weight loss. Although denying that she has a problem, she reveals that she became a vegetarian and stopped eating fat several months ago because she was heavier than the star of the track team. She thinks she still needs to lose some weight, but it has become much harder now. Recently she has felt exhausted and cold all the time, and is having trouble sleeping. She is worried that her grades are not good enough to get into a good college. In addition, she blacked out in the shower last week, and didn't tell her mother. A.N. denies sexual activity or drug use, and denies using self-induced vomiting or laxatives to control her weight. Her last normal period was over 5 months ago.

Based on the above history, you make a diagnosis of anorexia nervosa (AN), the third most common chronic condition of childhood behind asthma and obesity. AN is a psychiatric disorder characterized by an intense fear of becoming obese, disturbance in perception of one's body shape or size, the absence of at least three consecutive menstrual cycles in postmenarchal females, and refusal to maintain body weight above 15th percentile expected for age and height. Other common findings include excessive physical activity, preoccupation with food, and sleep and mood disturbances. Mortality is approximately 10%; the most common cause of death is suicide, followed by death from the cardiac complications of starvation, refeeding, or electrolyte imbalance.

Treatment is aimed at restoring nutritional balance to achieve weight gain, correcting physiologic abnormalities, and addressing the underlying psychiatric disturbance. Patients with electrolyte imbalance, abnormal vital signs, or cardiac rhythm disturbances should be admitted for inpatient management. Most treatment programs combine behavior modification and psychotherapy with medical and nutritional support. Success of treatment is estimated at 50% to 70%.

QUESTIONS

173. Bulimia nervosa is characterized by each the following *except*:
    A. Recurrent binge eating, with a fear of not being able to stop eating
    B. Purging of excessive intake with exercise, self-induced vomiting or cathartics
    C. Drastic weight loss
    D. Excessive concern over weight and body appearance

174. Consequences of anorexia nervosa may include which of the following:
    A. Cardiac arrhythmias
    B. Chronic inability to maintain normal weight
    C. Osteoporosis
    D. All of the above

175. Which of the following is *not* a part of the "female athlete triad"
    A. Amenorrhea
    B. Anorexia
    C. Osteoporosis
    D. Sports-related injuries

176. Anorexia nervosa occurs:
    A. In females only
    B. In all socioeconomic groups
    C. More commonly than bulimia nervosa
    D. In Caucasians only

ID/CC: 3 1/2-year-old boy is brought in by his mother for poor appetite and weight loss.

HPI: A.L. had been healthy until 3 to 4 weeks ago when he developed a fever and cough. At that time, his mother was told by the doctor that he had a virus, but she now reports that he has "never really recovered." Since then, he has been sleeping more than usual, and his appetite has been poor. Recently mother thinks he looks thin and pale, and she has noticed dark circles under his eyes. He has continued to have low-grade fevers, but has not had vomiting, diarrhea, abdominal pain, cough, or runny nose. He does not have any rashes, but mother thinks he is bruising more easily than before. Mother says his weight at his last visit 3 weeks ago was 35 lbs (16 kg).

PMHx: None   **Meds:** None

SHx: Parents are divorced, patient lives with mother. Two older brothers are healthy.

VS: Temp 37.7°C (99.8°F), BP 95/72, HR 105, RR 22; Weight 13.5 kg (25%)

PE: *Gen:* thin, tired-appearing, pale boy sitting in mother's lap. *HEENT:* mucous membranes are pale but moist, with pinpoint purple macules scattered on the buccal mucosa. TM and oropharynx clear, no nuchal rigidity. Nontender anterior and posterior lymphadenopathy is noted bilaterally, and nodes are palpable in the supraclavicular and occipital areas. *CV:* tachycardia with a soft flow murmur; otherwise, within normal limits. *Abdomen:* soft and nontender. Spleen tip palpable, liver edge felt 2 cm below the costal margin. *Skin:* pale, but warm and well-perfused. Several purplish bruises are noted over the shins, no petechiae or other rashes. Remainder of exam within normal limits.

THOUGHT QUESTIONS

- What is your differential diagnosis at this point?
- What further workup would you pursue?

A.L.'s weight loss and ill appearance suggest a chronic rather than an acute process. He has a constellation of nonspecific symptoms (i.e., fever, malaise, lymphadenopathy, hepatosplenomegaly, and pallor) that can be attributed to a large variety of diseases. In broad categories these include infection (e.g., viral infections such as EBV or HIV can present with these findings, as can subacute or chronic bacterial infections), rheumatologic disease (e.g., lupus or JRA often present with nonspecific systemic findings such as fever or weight loss in children), and malignancy. Malignancy is of particular concern in this child, as his pallor, mucosal petechiae, bruising, and fever suggest bone marrow dysfunction.

With the broad differential above, the first screening lab tests should be a CBC with differential. The CBC is a good indicator of infection or inflammation, as well as bone marrow function, and the results may guide further testing. Other blood tests to consider as indicated by examination and history in cases like this include an ESR or CRP, an ANA, blood cultures, and specific viral serologies.

CASE CONTINUED

You draw blood for a CBC which reveals a WBC of 3000, Hct of 23, and platelets of 57. The automated differential shows 86% lymphocytes and 10% neutrophils. Shortly thereafter, the laboratory calls because the manual differential reveals 5% blasts.

The findings on physical examination, along with the presence of pancytopenia on CBC and blasts on peripheral smear suggest acute lymphocytic leukemia (ALL), the most common malignancy diagnosed in children. You consult the oncology service and obtain a bone marrow biopsy, which confirms the diagnosis of ALL with 35% lymphoblasts present on bone marrow examination. A.L. is admitted for further laboratory tests and for the initiation of chemotherapy. Because of his young age, low initial lymphocyte count and lymphoid cell lineage, he falls into a favorable prognostic category, and is felt to have an excellent chance of full recovery.

Leukemias are the most common childhood malignancies, representing 25% to 30% of the malignancies diagnosed each year. CNS tumors, lymphoma, and neuroblastoma follow in frequency. About 97% of all childhood leukemias are acute, and 80% of these are lymphocytic. Presenting features include signs of bone marrow infiltration (e.g., pallor, bruising or petechiae, and fever or prolonged infection), bone or joint pain (caused by leukemic expansion of bone marrow cavity), lymphadenopathy, and weight loss. The diagnosis is suggested by peripheral blasts and evidence of bone marrow failure on CBC, and confirmed by bone marrow examination.

QUESTIONS

177. Treatment of ALL:
     A. Rarely results in a cure
     B. Can usually be accomplished as an outpatient
     C. Includes routine bone marrow transplant
     D. Must include management of complications at presentation, as well as those resulting from treatment

178. Which of the following are likely consequences of treatment of leukemia?
     A. Tumor lysis syndrome (hyperuricemia, hyperkalemia, and hyperphosphatemia)
     B. Severe bone marrow suppression
     C. Alopecia
     D. All of the above

179. Which of the following is true of brain tumors in children?
     A. They are the least common solid tumors of childhood.
     B. They are usually supratentorial (i.e., involving the cerebral hemispheres).
     C. They are usually infratentorial (i.e., involving the cerebellum, midbrain, and brainstem).
     D. Presentation is similar regardless of location.

180. Each of the following is true of lymphomas in children except:
     A. They account for 10% to 15% of all childhood cancers.
     B. Most cases are Hodgkin type.
     C. Peripheral blood counts are usually normal at presentation.
     D. Overall long-term survival rates are favorable.

ID/CC: 4-month-old boy is brought to the clinic with poor weight gain.

HPI: Mother was told that F.T. was not gaining weight at his last doctor's visit 2 weeks ago, and she is concerned that he still looks small. The baby is a good eater but spits up "all the time" and is difficult to feed. He has bowel movements three to four times per day, and his stool is greenish, liquid, and nonbloody. He urinates approximately four times per day (normal six to eight). F.T. cries only when he is hungry, and sleeps "great," sometimes almost the whole night. The infant has not had fever, cough, respiratory distress, vomiting, or diarrhea. He is developmentally normal.

PMHx: Normal birth history, full-term delivery without complications. Birth weight was 7 lbs, 10 oz (3460 gram, 60%). No hospitalizations or illnesses.

Meds: None   **All:** NKDA   **Immunizations:** UTD

VS: Temp 36.8°F, HR 130, RR 38; pO_2 = 99% on RA; Weight 5230 gram (10%), Length 65 cm (70%), Head circumference 43 cm (70%); Weight at last doctor's visit 2 weeks ago: 5190 gram (15%)

PE: *Gen:* somewhat fussy but consolable infant, who appears small for age. *HEENT:* nondysmorphic. Anterior fontanelle slightly sunken and soft. Mucus membranes moist, oropharynx clear without thrush, palate intact. *Lungs:* clear. *CV:* RR&R without murmur, pulses and cap refill brisk. *Abdomen:* soft, nontender with NABS, no epatosplenomegaly. *Neuro:* deep tendon reflexes and tone are normal; developmentally appropriate for age.

THOUGHT QUESTIONS

- Plot this infant on a growth chart. What are possible causes of poor growth in this infant?

- What additional information will you seek on history or examination, and what further workup would you like to obtain on this infant?

This child is not gaining weight as expected for his age, a condition known as failure to thrive (FTT). FTT is defined as a fall in weight to below the 3rd percentile for age, or a deceleration of growth crossing two major percentiles on a standard growth chart. The causes of FTT may be organic or nonorganic, or a combination of the two. Because the differential diagnosis is extensive, it is often helpful to divide it into causes of decreased intake and increased output. Decreased intake is usually an environmental issue, such as poverty, abuse or neglect, inexperienced parents, or poor bonding between infant and parent. Additionally, disease processes that can cause feeding difficulties must be considered, especially neurologic disorders and malformations of the mouth and palate. Causes of increased output are more likely to be organic in nature. These include malabsorption, metabolic disease, malignancy, chronic or acute infection, and endocrine disturbances.

The evaluation for failure to thrive should start with a careful history and physical examination. Details of feeding and output, as well as information on recent illnesses, developmental history, and family history of small stature or growth delay should be elicited. Of utmost importance is a detailed social history, including the infant's home environment, temperament, and any recent financial or social stressors present in the family. Laboratory studies should be ordered based on the likely cause of the FTT, and on concern for any metabolic derangements as a result of poor nutrition or intrinsic disease. Appropriate screening tests to consider include a CBC, electrolytes, and stool studies.

CASE CONTINUED

Further history reveals that mother is 16 years old, lives with her parents and attends high school, and has felt overwhelmed by the care of the child. F.T. takes a 4- to 6-oz bottle of formula every 3 hours during the day. He often spits up after feeds, and if he is still thirsty afterward she gives him water. During the night he rarely wakes to feed. You decide to observe the child feeding, and give mother a bottle of formula, which the infant takes vigorously, then spits up a small amount. You also send a stool guaiac, stool reducing substances, and pH, all of which are within normal limits.

THOUGHT QUESTION

• How would you manage this patient?

Based on F.T.'s normal physical examination and the history suggesting inadequate caloric intake due to infrequent feeds and supplementation with water, you suspect a nonorganic form of failure to thrive. There are several ways to manage this infant, and the proper management depends on the physician's impression of the family's ability and motivation to comply with outpatient treatment. Although hospitalization is necessary in cases of obvious or suspected neglect, in this case it would be reasonable to educate the mother on proper feeding of an infant this age, and if possible involve the grandparents as well in the education. Close follow-up by phone and weekly weight checks should be performed. If the infant fails to gain weight with adequate intake as an outpatient, he should be admitted to observe feeding in-house and to undertake further testing if growth does not respond as expected.

QUESTIONS

181. In most cases of FTT:
    A. The cause is organic.
    B. The cause is nonorganic.
    C. The cause is a combination of organic and nonorganic.
    D. The infant or child never achieves normal weight or growth.

182. Risk factors for FTT include each of the following *except*:
    A. Middle or high socioeconomic status
    B. History of prematurity or other neonatal problems
    C. Chronic disease
    D. Maternal depression

183. You should be more concerned about an organic cause of FTT if:
    A. The child gains weight when proper feeding is reinstated
    B. Head circumference and length are impaired as well as weight
    C. Laboratory tests are normal
    D. Physical examination is normal

184. An appropriate diet for a full term infant should include:
    A. Fresh fruits and vegetables
    B. Cow's milk
    C. Breast milk or formula only
    D. Water to drink between feeds

ID/CC: 7-year-old girl is brought to the clinic complaining of an itchy rash for 2 days.

HPI: S.F.'s rash started on the trunk and has spread to her back, arms, and thighs. Her mother has applied calamine lotion with modest relief. S.F. was kept home from school today because of a fever, and this morning refused to eat breakfast because of a stomachache. She also states that it hurts to swallow. There is no history of runny nose or cough, joint pain, chest pain, or dysuria. This is the first time she has had a rash.

PMHx: Never hospitalized, no surgeries   **Meds:** Calamine lotion, Tylenol for fever

All: NKDA   **Immunizations:** UTD

SHx: Has a new kitten at home. Plays goalie for her soccer team.

> ### THOUGHT QUESTIONS
> - What is your differential diagnosis?
> - What findings will you look for on physical examination, and which laboratory tests would you consider to help with your diagnosis?

The differential diagnosis should include a variety of bacterial and viral syndromes that can cause fever and rash, including adenovirus, mononucleosis, scarlet fever (group A *Streptococcus* pharyngitis), acute rheumatic fever, toxic shock syndrome, and sepsis. Other noninfectious entities that can cause this type of rash include Kawasaki syndrome, eczema, allergic or contact dermatitis, drug allergy, and anaphylaxis.

Your first priority, as always, should be to ensure that the patient is hemodynamically stable. In particular, toxic shock syndrome, sepsis, and anaphylaxis will cause hypotension and impending airway compromise, and it is important to identify them early. Physical examination should include careful documentation of the distribution and appearance of the rash, with subsequent focus on identification of the characteristic features of the above bacterial and viral syndromes, such as conjunctivitis, exudative pharyngitis, adenopathy, and arthritis. The use of laboratory tests should be guided by examination findings. Consider the rapid tests available for common infections such as mononucleosis and group A *Streptococcus*.

CASE CONTINUED

VS: Temp 39.5°C (103.2°F), BP 100/70, HR 120, RR 21; Weight 22 kg (40%)

PE: *Gen:* uncomfortable but nontoxic girl, appears generally healthy *HEENT:* the oropharynx is remarkable for enlarged, erythematous tonsils with exudate visible on the right. Enlarged, tender cervical lymph nodes are palpable bilaterally. The tongue appears pale with reddish, hypertrophic papillae. There is no conjunctivitis or rhinorrhea. *CV:* RR&R, no murmur, pulses equal, cap refill brisk *Skin:* diffuse, blanching, dry, finely papular, rough-feeling erythematous patches covering trunk, back, arms, thighs. Creases in the skin folds of the arms and groin appear enhanced. *Musculoskeletal:* MS: full ROM, no joint swelling or pain. Remainder of exam is within normal limits.

Labs: Rapid throat group A *Strep* screen positive. Mono spot negative. Throat culture pending.

THOUGHT QUESTIONS

- What is the most likely diagnosis?
- How would you treat this patient, and what long-term consequences are you attempting to prevent by treating her?

This patient has *scarlet fever,* a syndrome consisting of group A *Streptococcus* (GAS) pharyngitis with a toxin-mediated rash. The rash is typically a diffuse, dry, sandpaper-like pruritic rash that starts on the trunk or neck and spreads to the extremities. It is more pronounced in skin creases, a finding known as Pastia's lines.

GAS pharyngitis typically presents as a triad of pharyngitis, lymphadenopathy, and fever. Stomach pain, headache, or an associated rash may also be present, but upper respiratory infection symptoms are notably absent. Diagnosis is made by throat culture. In addition to the pharynx, GAS may infect the skin, the urine, or the lymph nodes (adenitis). Although usually self-limited, GAS infections can result in both suppurative (e.g., peritonsillar abscess, retropharyngeal abscess) and non-suppurative (e.g., acute rheumatic fever [ARF], acute poststreptococcal glomerulonephritis [PSGN]) consequences. Treatment with penicillin is universally recommended to prevent ARF, although it has *not* been shown to shorten duration or severity of symptoms or prevent PSGN.

QUESTIONS

185. Which of the following is considered the gold standard for diagnosis of GAS pharyngitis?
    A. Clinical exam
    B. Rapid antigen test
    C. Throat culture
    D. Response to treatment

186. Each of the following are considered major criteria for the diagnosis of acute rheumatic fever *except*:
    A. Polyarthritis
    B. Subcutaneous nodules
    C. Carditis
    D. Positive culture for group A streptococci

187. Poststreptococcal glomerulonephritis most often occurs after GAS infection of:
    A. The pharynx
    B. The skin
    C. The urine
    D. The blood

188. Toxic shock syndrome is usually the result of a toxin produced by which bacteria?
    A. Group A streptococci
    B. *Neisseria meningitidis*
    C. *Staphylococcus aureus*
    D. *Staphylococcus epidermidis*

ID/CC: 7-year-old boy is brought in by his father for a rash.

HPI: I.T.'s rash started 2 days ago with some red dots around the eyes. It has now spread to the chest and back, and is starting to appear on his arms and legs as well. The rash is not itchy or painful, and I.T. has never had a rash like this before. Although he recently got over a cold, I.T. has been feeling completely well, without fever, cough, sore throat, headache, neck stiffness, nausea, or vomiting. In fact, he is mad at his father for making him come to see the doctor.

PMHx: None   **Meds:** None   **All:** NKDA   **Immunizations:** UTD

SHx: Parents are divorced, lives with father. No significant family illnesses.

VS: Temp 37.2°C (98.9°F), BP 100/65, HR 92, RR 19; Weight 25 kg (65%)

PE: *Gen:* sullen but cooperative boy, in no acute distress, wearing a Limp Bizkit T-shirt *HEENT:* good dentition, clear oropharynx except for a small amount of oozing blood around the gums. Nares are clear. No nuchal rigidity or photophobia. No lymphadenopathy. *Abdomen:* soft, nontender, no masses, no hepatosplenomegaly. *Skin:* multiple discrete, smooth, nonblanching pinpoint (1 to 2 mm) red-purple macules diffusely cover the face, chest and back, they are also seen on arms and legs. There is no scale or excoriation on the rash. A few 3- to 4-cm areas of subcutaneous bluish discoloration are noted on the child's legs. Remainder of exam is within normal limits.

THOUGHT QUESTIONS

- What is the name of this type of rash, and what are some of its likely causes?
- What further history would you like to obtain, and what laboratory tests would you request to help with the diagnosis?

This well-appearing patient has a diffuse petechial rash, characterized by scattered discrete purple or red nonblanching pinpoint macules. This type of rash may have many causes, some of which are benign, and others that are immediately life-threatening. If at any time a patient with this rash appears toxic or hemodynamically unstable, sepsis is presumed and the patient should be stabilized with fluid resuscitation and antibiotics immediately. In the nontoxic, stable child a more leisurely search for the likely cause can be performed.

Petechiae are usually caused by an alteration in the number or function of platelets. In general, platelets can be affected by infection, malignancy, autoimmune processes, and consumption by the spleen. Because the differential diagnoses is so wide, the history and physical examination are key in identifying accompanying symptoms such as fever, headache, irritability, other types of bleeding (especially mucosal bleeding, epistaxis, or hematuria), organomegaly, joint swelling or pain, malaise, weight loss, and a recent history of medication or drug use. The most important screening test in evaluating a petechial rash is the CBC, which enumerates platelets as well as other cell lines that may indicate infection or bone marrow failure. A PT and partial thromboplastin time (PTT) are also helpful, especially when the CBC reveals a normal platelet number; a blood culture should be sent as well.

CASE CONTINUED

There is no history of easy bruising, bleeding or joint pain, or swelling. I.T. notes that his gums bled a bit when he brushed his teeth this morning. He denies recent use of antibiotics, aspirin, or other medications.

Labs: CBC: WBC of 7.6 with normal differential, hematocrit: 38. Platelets 12,000. Smear reveals giant platelets (megakaryocytes); otherwise normal morphology. Coags normal (PT 13.6, PTT 37.5). Blood culture sent.

THOUGHT QUESTION

- What is your diagnosis, based on the examination and laboratory findings?

Given this patient's well appearance and profound thrombocytopenia, without additional laboratory abnormalities, he is diagnosed with idiopathic thrombocytopenic purpura (ITP). ITP, also known as immune thrombocytopenic purpura, is the most common cause of thrombocytopenia in children. It results from the binding of antiplatelet antibodies to platelet membranes, followed by their destruction by the reticuloendothelial system; it often occurs several weeks after a viral illness. Patients are completely well-appearing, and aside from an often profound thrombocytopenia, laboratory tests including CBC, coagulation studies, and blood culture should all be normal.

QUESTIONS

189. Management of this patient should include all of the following *except*:
    A. Platelet transfusion
    B. Avoidance of contact sports
    C. Treatment with IV steroids or IVIG until platelet count begins to recover
    D. Regular outpatient checks of platelet count to document recovery

190. If this patient had been unstable or toxic-appearing, which antibiotic(s) would you start *immediately* (while initiating vigorous fluid resuscitation and obtaining blood and CSF cultures)?
    A. Erythromycin
    B. Ceftriaxone
    C. Ceftriaxone and vancomycin
    D. Ampicillin and gentamicin

191. Chronic ITP is defined as persistent thrombocytopenia for:
    A. 2 to 4 weeks
    B. 1 to 2 months
    C. 6 to 12 months
    D. Longer than 1 year

192. Henoch-Schönlein purpura (HSP), one of the conditions in the differential diagnosis for this case, is associated with all of the following findings *except*:
    A. Purpuric or petechial rash on buttocks and legs
    B. Heart murmur
    C. Abdominal pain
    D. Joint pain

ID/CC: 5-year-old boy is brought in by his father for a rash and swelling around his left eye.

HPI: The swelling was noted early this morning before school, and this afternoon it seemed to be getting worse. P.C. complains of itching and discomfort around the eye, but has no difficulty with vision. He has no fever, runny nose, or malaise. P.C. and his father deny trauma to the eye, but there was a mosquito bite on the left cheek a few days ago that was very itchy, and his father worries that it might have become infected. He says, "I told him to stop scratching it."

PMHx: No hospitalizations, no medication allergies, hayfever in the spring.

Meds: None   **All:** NKDA   **Immunizations:** UTD

SHx: P.C. is in kindergarten, plays third base for his T-ball team.

THOUGHT QUESTIONS

- What diagnosis are you most concerned about in this patient?
- What examination findings will you specifically look for, and which, if any, laboratory tests would you consider?

The most important diagnosis to exclude is orbital cellulitis, a dangerous infection that involves the tissues behind the orbit and is often hematogenous in origin. Orbital cellulitis, which by definition extends posterior to the orbital septum and thus endangers vision, is a medical emergency. It is characterized by an abrupt onset of severe eye swelling with proptosis and limitation of extraocular movement, and occasionally by visual impairment. Systemic toxicity is common, especially in infants. In contrast, periorbital or preseptal cellulitis is a limited infection that does not cause these findings.

A careful examination of the eye and its movements is essential with any eye swelling to guide further investigation. If orbital cellulitis is suspected, blood cultures should be drawn and the child should be admitted for close observation and IV antibiotics selected to cover the most likely organisms, including *Haemophilus influenzae* type B and *Streptococcus pneumoniae*. Imaging should be performed to delineate involvement of the orbital tissues or sinuses, and to rule out complications such as orbital abscess or brain abscess. Cultures should be sent of nearby skin lesions as well as CSF, and an ophthalmology consultation should be obtained.

CASE CONTINUED

VS: Temp 37.1°C (98.7°F), BP 110/70, HR 110, RR 20; Weight 18 kg (50%)

PE: *Gen:* alert, nontoxic appearing, well-developed boy in no acute distress. *HEENT:* left upper eyelid mildly swollen and slightly erythematous, with extension of pink color to left upper cheekbone and around a yellow-crusted insect bite. The skin is tender to palpation around the insect bite, and slightly warm to the touch. Extraocular movements (EOMs) are intact without pain, and no proptosis or scleral injection is noted. Visual acuity is 20/20 in both eyes. There is no sinus tenderness, TMs are normal bilaterally, oropharynx is clear, and no lymphadenopathy is noted. The teeth appear healthy, no cavities are visible. Remainder of exam within normal limits.

THOUGHT QUESTIONS

- What is your differential and most likely diagnosis?
- How would you manage this patient?

The differential diagnosis for this well-appearing young man with periorbital swelling and a nearby crusted lesion includes periorbital cellulitis, conjunctivitis, an allergic reaction, angioedema, varicella virus infection (chickenpox or zoster) or cellulitis extending from infection of the sinuses, teeth, or other facial structures. Of these, the most likely diagnosis is early periorbital cellulitis without evidence of orbital involvement. He also seems to have an early superinfection, or impetigo, of his insect bite.

Cellulitis is a bacterial infection of the skin characterized by redness, warmth, and tenderness. It is usually caused by the skin's normal flora (e.g., group A β-hemolytic *Streptococcus, Staphylococcus aureus*) gaining access to the dermis and epidermis through a break in the integument (like the insect bite). Treatment of localized cellulitis in a nontoxic appearing child can be accomplished on an outpatient basis with an appropriate oral antibiotic active against staphylococcal and strepto-coccal species (e.g., cephalexin or amoxicillin/clavulanic acid are good choices). An antihistamine will help with itching, and an oral pain reliever with discomfort. It is also helpful to draw a line around the erythematous area in the clinic, so that the patient or parent can monitor carefully for any further spread of the infection. Any cellulitis that is associated with fever, toxicity, rapid spread, or lymphangitic streaking should be treated with intravenous antibiotics, such as oxacillin, and a blood culture should be performed to rule out bacteremia.

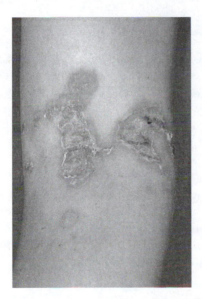

FIGURE 49 Typical appearance of impetigo. Used with permission from Rudolf M, Levene M. Paediatrics and Child Health. Oxford: Blackwell Science, Ltd., 1999: 209.

QUESTIONS

193. Facial cellulitis can be a sign of each of the following underlying infections *except*:
    A. Bacteremia
    B. Sinusitis
    C. Dental infection
    D. Meningitis

194. This child's insect bite is most likely superinfected with:
    A. *Staphylococcus* species
    B. *Streptococcus* species
    C. Gram-negative organisms
    D. *Pseudomonas* species

195. Each of the following would raise concern for an early anaphylactic reaction in this patient *except*:
    A. Fever
    B. Hypotension
    C. Lip or tongue swelling
    D. Wheeze

196. Which of the following is *not* a finding in conjunctivitis ("pink eye")?
    A. Conjunctival and scleral injection
    B. Eye pruritus
    C. Eye discharge
    D. Severe eye pain

ID/CC: A 2.5-year-old girl is brought in by her father for an itchy rash for 2 weeks.

HPI: The rash first appeared on A.D.'s neck, and now has spread to her face, hands, and trunk. Recently, A.D. has been awake and scratching at night, making the rash worse, and her father is worried that it has become infected on one of her hands. She has always had dry, sensitive skin, which has been worse this winter. She developed a similar rash a few months ago after playing on a neighbor's lawn, but has been otherwise well, without fever or malaise.

MPHx: A.D. tends to wheeze when she gets a cold, and father was told she had something called "reactive airway disease." Never hospitalized, no surgeries, no recent illnesses.

Meds: None **All:** NKDA **Immunizations:** UTD

FHx: 6-year-old brother has asthma. Mother has "dry skin" on her eyelids and hands, is allergic to strawberries and gets "horrible hayfever" in the spring.

THOUGHT QUESTIONS

• What is the differential diagnosis?

• What details about the rash will you ask about in further history and look for when you examine the child to help in your diagnosis?

The differential diagnosis in this case includes a variety of allergic and infectious rashes, in particular atopic dermatitis, contact dermatitis, rhus dermatitis (poison oak or poison ivy), psoriasis, seborrheic dermatitis, ringworm, scabies, and impetigo. With most dermatologic conditions, the history and examination are the keys to diagnosis. You should discern the physical and temporal pattern of the rash, as well as its relation to any possible infectious or environmental triggers such as insects, plants or pollen, food, pets, stress, sunlight, household chemicals, or allergens.

CASE CONTINUED

On further history, the rash does not seem to be related to any particular foods, although A.D. eats "everything." There have not been any new detergents, soaps, or lotions used on the child or her clothes. The family lives in an apartment in the city, and they have a 2-year-old dog and a new parakeet. There are no smokers at home, although several of the parents' friends smoke. The family has not traveled out of the state and has not been hiking or camping recently.

VS: Temp 36.9°C (98.4°F), HR 120, RR 28; Weight 15 kg (85%)

PE: *Gen:* well-appearing and playful little girl, scratching at her left hand and belly. *HEENT:* mild rhinorrhea, pale nasal mucosa, otherwise normal. *Skin:* patches of dry, papular skin are noted behind the ears, at the nape of the neck, and behind the knees. Areas of red, papular, excoriated skin are present on flexor surfaces of both wrists and cheeks, as well as on the trunk. There are no vesicles or burrows seen, and the diaper area is notably free of rash. The left wrist has several deep excoriations, some coated with a golden crust. Remainder of exam is within normal limits.

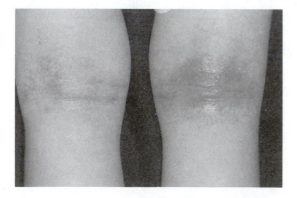

FIGURE 50 Rash on extensor surfaces of legs, as might be seen on this patient. Used with permission from Rudolf M, Levene M. Paediatrics and Child Health. Oxford: Blackwell Science, Ltd., 1999: 203.

THOUGHT QUESTIONS

• What is your diagnosis?

• How would you manage this patient?

This child has atopic dermatitis, or eczema. Atopic dermatitis is a common allergic skin condition that affects about 5% of children before the age of 5, with the majority (60%) developing the condition before the age of 1 year. The morphology and distribution of the rash changes with age: infants 2 months to 2 years have weeping, pruritic patches on the face, scalp, trunk, and extremities; older children have erythematous, excoriated papular patches on the flexor surfaces of extremities and backs of hands and feet; adolescents and adults have dry, scaly patches on the hands and feet, flexor surfaces, and eyelids.

Treatment of eczema involves both alleviation of current symptoms and prevention of subsequent flares, which increase the risk of infection and permanent scarring. Management of acute flares should include application of topical steroids, control of itching to prevent scratching, and moisturization of the skin. Superficial infection with *Staphylococcus* is common, and a topical antibiotic, such as Bactroban, may be applied to these areas. The patient should minimize exposure to pets and to any known food allergens, as well as to soaps, lotions, and detergents that contain fragrances and irritating chemicals. Referral to a dermatologist or allergist may be necessary in severe or refractory cases.

QUESTIONS

197. The cause of eczema is:
     A. Pollution
     B. Poor hygiene
     C. Early exposure to synthetic chemicals
     D. Unknown

198. Each of the following would be helpful in reducing symptoms for a child with eczema *except*:
     A. Bathing in hot water and scrubbing vigorously with soap
     B. An oral antihistamine at bedtime
     C. Trimming fingernails short
     D. Emollient lotion applied immediately after bathing, and regularly throughout the day

199. Which of the following skin disorders in the differential diagnosis for this case is characterized by annular patches with central clearing and a scaly border?
     A. Scabies
     B. Seborrheic dermatitis
     C. Ringworm
     D. Psoriasis

200. All of the following are true of topical steroid therapy *except*:
     A. Thinning of the skin may occur with prolonged use.
     B. Growth retardation is common.
     C. Application should be avoided in delicate areas such as the eyelids and genitals.
     D. Agents of various potencies are available.

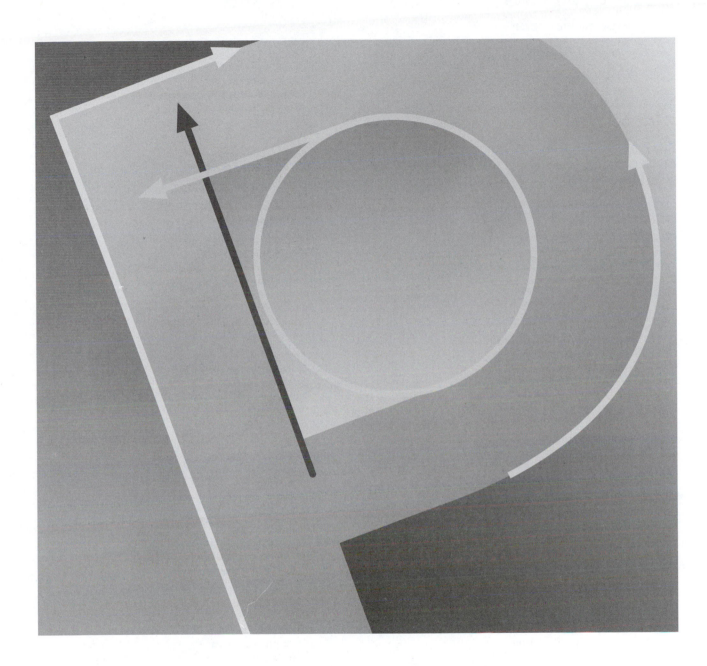

ANSWERS

CASE PRESENTATIONS

CASES PRESENTING WITH FEVER
Case 1. Fever and Fussiness
Case 2. Fever and Vomiting
Case 3. Febrile Infant
Case 4. Fever and Adenopathy
Case 5. High Fever
Case 6. Fever and Irritability

CASES PRESENTING WITH RESPIRATORY DISTRESS
Case 7. Infant with Cough
Case 8. Wheezing
Case 9. Cough and Runny Nose
Case 10. Persistent Shortness of Breath
Case 11. Wheezing and Rash
Case 12. Cough and Fever
Case 13. Persistent Cough

CASES IN A NEWBORN PATIENT
Case 14. Yellow Newborn
Case 15. Tachypneic Premature Newborn
Case 16. Cyanotic Newborn
Case 17. Bilious Vomiting
Case 18. Rapid Heart Rate
Case 19. Ambiguous Genitalia

CASES PRESENTING WITH ABDOMINAL PAIN
Case 20. Fever and Abdominal Pain
Case 21. Abdominal Pain and Vomiting
Case 22. Scrotal Pain and Swelling
Case 23. Infant with Indigestion
Case 24. Abdominal Pain and Bloody Diarrhea
Case 25. Cramps and Watery Diarrhea

CASES PRESENTING WITH VOMITING
Case 26. Vomiting and Diarrhea
Case 27. Vomiting Infant
Case 28. Vomiting and Irritability
Case 29. Vomiting Blood

CASES PRESENTING WITH JOINT PAIN
Case 30. Hip Pain
Case 31. Knee Pain
Case 32. Shoulder Pain
Case 33. Puffy Hands and Feet

CASES PRESENTING WITH REFUSAL TO WALK
Case 34. Limping Teen
Case 35. Difficulty Walking
Case 36. Never Started Walking
Case 37. Sore Foot and Dark Urine
Case 38. Febrile Toddler

CASES PRESENTING WITH ALTERED MENTAL STATUS
Case 39. Seizure
Case 40. Shock
Case 41. Irritability
Case 42. Confusion After a Fall
Case 43. Erratic Behavior

CASES PRESENTING WITH WEIGHT LOSS
Case 44. Teen with Poor Appetite
Case 45. Weight Loss and Pallor
Case 46. Small Infant

CASES PRESENTING WITH A RASH
Case 47. Rash and Sore Throat
Case 48. Painless Dots
Case 49. Periorbital Redness
Case 50. Itchy Rash

DIAGNOSIS

Otitis Media
Urinary Tract Infection (UTI)
Occult Bacteremia
Epstein-Barr Virus
Coxsackie Virus A (Hand-Foot-Mouth Disease)
Acute Bacterial Meningitis

Croup
Foreign Body Aspiration
Bacterial Pneumonia
Asthma Exacerbation
Anaphylaxis
Bronchiolitis
Cystic Fibrosis

Physiologic Jaundice
Respiratory Distress Syndrome (RDS)
Transposition of Great Arteries
Malrotation/Volvulus
Supraventricular Tachycardia
Congenital Adrenal Hyperplasia

Appendicitis
Diabetic Ketoacidosis (DKA)
Testicular Torsion
Epilepsy
Inflammatory Bowel Disease
Dehydration

Viral Gastroenteritis
Pyloric Stenosis
Intussusception
GI Bleed

Toxic Synovitis
Juvenile Rheumatoid Arthritis (JRA)
Radial Head Subluxation (Nursemaid's Elbow)
Sickle Cell Disease

Slipped Capital Femoral Epiphysis (SCFE)
Guillain-Barre
Developmental Delay/Lead Poisoning
Glomerulonephritis
Osteomyelitis

Febrile Seizure
Viral Myocarditis
Child Abuse
Epidural Hematoma
Toxic Ingestion

Anorexia Nervosa
Acute Lymphocytic Leukemia (ALL)
Failure to Thrive

Scarlet Fever
Idiopathic Thrombocytopenic Purpura (ITP)
Periorbital Cellulitis
Eczema (Atoptic Dermatitis)

1–A

Ear pits, a congenital anomaly consisting of tiny holes anterior to the tragus that are occasionally associated with renal anomalies, are *not* a complication of otitis media. Mastoiditis, perforated TM, and chronic otitis are all complications of otitis media. Mastoiditis, an infection of the mastoid air cells, is characterized by posterior auricular swelling over the mastoid process, which may displace the ear laterally. It is a potentially serious infection that should be treated with parenteral antibiotics, and imaging should be considered to document the extent of the infection. A perforated TM usually does not require specific treatment; in fact, perforation is often accomplished intentionally in cases of chronic or recurrent otitis by the insertion of tympanostomy tubes. Chronic otitis, caused by anatomic predisposition to middle ear effusion or difficult to treat organisms, can be managed by the insertion of tubes, or by prophylactic antibiotic therapy. Other rare but serious complications of otitis media include meningitis, brain abscess, and lateral sinus thrombosis.

2–C

Hearing loss is usually reversible with relief of negative pressure within the middle ear. If it is significant and occurs during the years in which language is developing, it may affect language acquisition and cognitive development. It is the most prevalent complication of otitis media.

3–B

In the case of an otherwise healthy child with an otitis recurring despite recent antibiotic therapy, medication failure is most likely due to a resistant strain of *S. pneumoniae*. High-dose amoxicillin (60–80 mg/kg per day) has been shown to be effective against most drug-resistant strains of *S. pneumoniae*. Amoxicillin-clavulanic acid is a more expensive alternative that gives added coverage against *H. influenzae* and *M. catarrhalis*. If a child shows signs of systemic toxicity or intracranial spread of infection, admission and tympanocentesis for diagnostic purposes would be indicated. Polysporin otic drops are effective treatment for otitis externa, but are not indicated in otitis media.

4–A

Breastfeeding is actually considered a protective factor against otitis media. Day-care attendance, chronic middle ear effusion, and caretaker smoking are all recognized risk factors for otitis media.

Bottle-feeding, especially in the horizontal position, is another risk factor. Other risk factors include lower socioeconomic status, male gender, and Native American or Eskimo ethnicity.

5–B

A renal ultrasound should be performed on this patient to evaluate for hydronephrosis or urinary tract anomalies that could lead to further UTIs or renal damage. Most clinicians will consider imaging for the first UTI in any nonadolescent boy and in any girl under 2 years of age. Imaging is also considered in the setting of recurrent UTIs in all boys and nonadolescent girls. Any positive findings on ultrasound should be followed by a voiding cystourethrogram (VCUG) to further characterize urinary reflux or valve abnormalities. An IVP is not a useful study for identifying reflux or urinary tract abnormalities. Prophylactic antibiotics would be indicated if reflux is documented by one of the above studies.

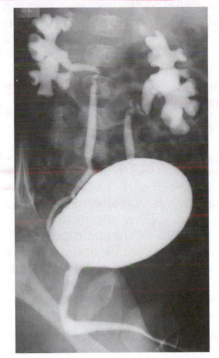

FIGURE A5 Severe bilateral vesicoureteric reflux on VCUG. Used with permission from Rudolf M, Levene M. Paediatrics and Child Health. Oxford: Blackwell Science, Ltd., 1999: 113.

6–B

Circumcision is actually considered protective against UTIs, and uncircumcised boys have a slightly higher risk of UTI. However, this is generally not considered sufficient to justify recommending circumcision for medical reasons. UTIs are 10 times more common in girls, although in infants younger than 1 year the prevalence is more or less equal for boys and girls. Other risk factors include a urinary tract abnormality that causes stasis, obstruction, or reflux, and instrumentation of the urethra or bladder.

7–D

Signs of UTI on urinalysis include leukocyte esterase, nitrites, and blood. The microscopy should show white cells and sometimes red cells present, as well as bacteria. It is important to keep in mind that in young infants these findings may not be present, as babies empty their bladders so quickly that the urine may not accumulate sufficient white cells or nitrites (which are produced by certain bacteria) to turn the test positive. Whenever a urinalysis suggests UTI, and in a febrile infant regardless of urinalysis results, a urine culture should be sent to confirm the diagnosis. A catheter specimen is always preferable for this purpose, because it is less likely to contain contamination with bacteria or white cells found on the perineum that can affect the urinalysis and culture. However, in older children it is reasonable to obtain a clean catch specimen first, to avoid the trauma of bladder catheterization, then to consider catheterization if the urinalysis reveals numerous epithelial cells, suggesting contamination.

8–C

The possible complications of UTI include renal scarring and abscesses in addition to renal failure. These consequences are rare in isolated bladder infections, but increase in likelihood with recurrence and severity of infection, as well as with the presence of anatomic abnormalities. Ureterocele is an anatomic abnormality that may predispose an individual to UTI but is not a consequence of UTI. Because of the risk of recurrent and damaging UTI in children with urinary tract abnormalities and urinary reflux, current guidelines recommend consideration of imaging to screen for these problems in selected populations. Ultrasound is generally performed first to identify hydronephrosis or gross anatomic abnormalities, followed several weeks after recovery by a VCUG (voiding cystourethrogram) to document the presence of urinary reflux. A nuclear study, the 2,3-dimercaptosuccinic acid (DMSA) scan, can be performed to document the presence of renal scarring in high-risk patients. Patients with documented reflux or anatomic abnormalities should be treated with prophylactic antibiotics and referred to a urologist for further management.

9–A

The most likely organisms recovered from blood cultures in well-appearing infants with occult bacteremia are *S. pneumoniae*, *H. influenzae* type b, and *N. meningitidis*. Currently, *S. pneumoniae* accounts for the vast majority of cases, although its prevalence may change due to the recent initiation of routine vaccination of children older than 2 months of age against this organism. In neonates (less than 1 month of age) with bacteremia or sepsis, Group B *Streptococcus*, *E. coli*, and *L. monocytogenes* are the organisms most often recovered from blood cultures. Most cases of occult bacteremia with *S. pneumoniae* resolve spontaneously in 24 to 48 hours, but there is a 3% risk of developing meningitis.

10–D

No particular ethnic, geographic, or socioeconomic factor has been found to correlate with higher risk of occult bacteremia. The other characteristics, including abnormally high or low WBC count, age <2 years, and high fever are all associated with an increased risk of occult bacteremia.

11–C

Sepsis is defined as an invasion of the intravascular compartment by bacteria. This invasion results in excessive release of endogenous mediators, leading to the clinical features of sepsis: circulatory collapse (shock) and multiorgan system involvement. Blood cultures often remain negative, and the absence of a causative organism should not preclude the diagnosis. High fever and elevated white blood cell count often accompany sepsis, but they also occur in occult bacteremia and many viral infections. Sepsis is a medical emergency, and it must be identified and treated early to prevent mortality. It is important to keep in mind that children often compensate well for early shock with tachycardia and vasoconstriction, so the appearance of these signs in a febrile or ill-appearing child should alert the clinician to the possibility of sepsis. The most common causes of sepsis in the child 3 to 36 months of age are the same as those responsible for occult bacteremia.

12–B

The presence of red cells is common in CSF obtained by lumbar puncture, and does not alone suggest bacterial meningitis. Bloody CSF that does not clear, however, should raise suspicion for a subarachnoid bleed or certain viral meningitides. The presence of white cells (>1 per 500 red cells), elevated protein, and decreased glucose in the CSF are all considered signs of meningitis, a diagnosis that is supported by culture of the CSF for bacteria or virus.

13–C

Brain abscess is *not* a known complication of mononucleosis, but cases of encephalitis, cerebellitis, and cranial neuritis have been reported. Complications of EBV infection are relatively common, but most are transient and relatively benign. Airway obstruction, a rare but serious complication, is of particular concern in young children, as their already small airways are more susceptible to obstruction by swollen pharyngeal tissue. Hematologic complications, which include neutropenia, thrombocytopenia, and hemolytic anemia, are quite common, and are usually transient. Steroids have been shown to be helpful in treating hematologic and obstructive complications. Splenic rupture is a rare but serious complication of EBV or CMV infection, so contact sports should be avoided as a preventive measure in patients with an enlarged or tender spleen. Hepatitis, usually asymptomatic with elevated transaminases, is another common but usually transient complication. Immunosuppressed individuals, especially after transplant surgery, are at risk of reactivation of dormant EBV, which contributes to lymphoproliferative disorder.

14–A

Diagnosis of mononucleosis is often made clinically, but can be supported by laboratory evaluation. The classic symptom triad includes fever, lymphadenopathy, and exudative pharyngitis. Occasional findings include an enlarged and tender spleen, and a maculopapular rash, which may occur spontaneously or after treatment with amoxicillin. Typical findings on CBC include a characteristic pattern of lymphocytosis, with up to 20% atypical lymphocytes; the remainder of the CBC is usually normal. The Monospot is a rapid test for antibodies against EBV, which is based on their interaction with heterophile cells (usually sheep red blood cells). The test is quite specific, but not very sensitive, and is most accurate after several weeks of infection. If the Monospot is negative, specific antibody tests including anti-EBV or anti-CMV IgM and IgG can be sent, especially if there is a question of chronic infection. Lymph node biopsy is

rarely indicated in the otherwise healthy child, and splenomegaly, present about 50% to 85% of the time in EBV infection, is not considered diagnostic.

15–B

Unilateral suppurative adenitis in young children is usually bacterial in origin, and the most common organisms are *Staphylococcus aureus* and *Streptococcus pyogenes*. Infection by *S. aureus*, the most common cause of adenitis in neonates and children under 4, is particularly likely to cause early suppuration, and is often preceded by a history of upper respiratory infection. In older children, anaerobes (often arising from dental or periodontal disease) and mycobacteria, as well as toxoplasmosis and catscratch disease, become the more likely organisms. Suspected staphylococcal or streptococcal adenitis in a nontoxic child should be treated with a course of oral first-generation cephalosporin, such as cephalexin, or another antibiotic with good staphylococcal and streptococcal coverage. Incision and drainage may be necessary if the node is very large or does not respond to appropriate oral therapy.

16–B

Strep throat, or group A *Streptococcus* pharyngitis, is a common cause of acute adenopathy but should not cause chronic adenopathy. Acute lymphocytic leukemia (ALL) is the most common malignancy of childhood, and often presents with painless, generalized lymphadenopathy. Although anterior cervical adenopathy is common in children, adenopathy that is painless, diffuse, hard, and located particularly in the posterior cervical triangle (where up to 50% of masses are malignant) should raise particular concern for malignancy. Tuberculosis and other mycobacteria, which often cause extrapulmonary disease in children, are a cause of subacute or chronic adenopathy. Occasionally mycobacteria cause a localized adenitis known as scrofula. Catscratch disease, a regional adenopathy sometimes accompanied by fever and systemic symptoms, is caused by *Bartonella henselae*. Cats are the common reservoir for this bacteria, and most patients have a recent history of contact with cats. Treatment is mainly supportive, as the disease is usually self-limited.

17–D

Antivirals are not effective against coxsackie virus infections. Although the disease is usually self-limited, dehydration from refusing to drink is likely. Pain and fever control, and ensuring adequate hydration are the mainstays of management. Oral antipyretics/analgesics such as acetaminophen or ibuprofen are useful, but aspirin should be avoided due to the association between viral illnesses and Reye syndrome. Some practitioners prescribe a mixture of Benadryl, Maalox, and viscous lidocaine ("magic mouthwash"), which may be swabbed onto the mouth prior to feeding to help with pain. Parents should encourage hydration with cool liquids and soft foods, and be taught how to identify signs of dehydration.

18–D

Parvovirus B19 (i.e., erythema infectiosum, slap-cheek rash, fifth disease) is a usually mild viral syndrome consisting of a low-grade fever followed by a rash that evolves in three stages. The first stage is marked erythema of the cheeks (a slapped-cheek appearance), which may be accompanied by circumoral pallor. The second is a maculopapular rash that begins on the arms and spreads to the trunk and legs, and may take on a reticulated or livedo appearance. The third stage lasts several weeks and consists of fluctuations in the appearance and severity of the rash, often in relation to light or heat exposure. Although self-limited in healthy children, parvovirus infections may cause a hemolytic anemia, which can precipitate an aplastic crisis in patients with sickle cell disease, and cause fetal hydrops if acquired during pregnancy.

Human herpesvirus 6 (i.e., HHV-6, roseola, exanthem subitum, sixth disease), one of the most common viral exanthems of childhood, consists of a prodrome of 1 to 5 days of high fever, followed on day 3 to 4 by a rose-colored macular rash that begins on the trunk and spreads to the periphery. Appearance of the rash is accompanied by resolution of the fever. The illness is benign, but may be associated with febrile seizures, due to the rapid rise of the fever.

Measles (rubeola) virus causes a clinical syndrome that occurs in three stages: 1) *Prodrome* consists of fever and the three Cs (cough, coryza, conjunctivitis). 2) *Koplik spots* (pathognomonic, white, 1- to 2-mm macules on an erythematous base), often with bluish flecks, are found on the buccal mucosa 2 to 3 days after the onset of fever, and 2 days before the rash. 3) *Rash*, which starts on the forehead or behind the ears, consists of discrete erythematous papules that coalesce and spread downward, lasting 6 to 7 days

and potentially undergoing desquamation. Although measles is now uncommon in the United States due to vaccination practices, sporadic epidemics still occur. The illness is usually self-limited, but complications include pneumonia, laryngitis, myocarditis, pericarditis, and thrombocytopenic purpura.

19–D

Varicella (i.e., chickenpox, zoster) is generally a self-limited viral infection in healthy toddlers. Treatment with acyclovir is recommended for newborns and teenagers as well as immunocompromised children, as these groups are at risk for more severe infection and complications. Although chickenpox infection was previously a rite of childhood, the recent initiation of widespread vaccination against the virus in the United States will likely impact its incidence. Clinically, infection with the virus is followed in 7 to 10 days by a mild fever and malaise, accompanied by crops of characteristic pruritic vesicles, beginning on the trunk and spreading peripherally. The lesions begin as red papules, develop a clear vesicle with a "teardrop on a rose petal" appearance, and then become cloudy, break, and become excoriated to form crusts or scabs. Lesions in various stages of development are typically present. The vesicles may occur on mucous membranes as well, including the cornea. Patients are infectious from 24 hours prior to the onset of the rash until all of the lesions are crusted. Possible complications of varicella include pneumonia, superinfection of the skin, and, in immunocompromised children, meningoencephalitis and systemic disease.

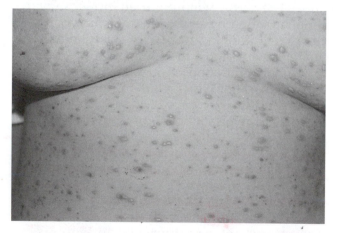

FIGURE A19 Typical vesicular rash of varicella infection. Used with permission from Banniser B, Begg N, Gillespie S. Infectious Disease, 2nd ed. Oxford: Blackwell Science, Ltd., 2000: plate 11.10.

20–C

Vomiting is *not* a part of the criteria for Kawasaki syndrome. The disease is a medium-vessel vasculitis of unclear etiology, diagnosed clinically by the presence of fever for more than 4 days, and four of five additional criteria (rash, mucus membrane involvement, unilateral cervical adenopathy, nonpurulent conjunctivitis, and swollen hands and feet). The primary morbidity of Kawasaki syndrome is its cardiac complications, which include coronary vasculitis and aneurysm formation leading to arrhythmias, infarction, congestive heart failure, and even death. Treatment of the syndrome with high-dose aspirin and 1 to 2 days of intravenous immunoglobulin (IVIG) significantly reduces the risk of coronary artery aneurysms.

21–A

The most common bacterial causes of meningitis in the infant or child are *S. pneumoniae*, *N. meningitidis*, and *H. influenzae.* Immunizations for all three exist, but only *H. influenzae* and *S. pneumoniae* are part of the routine immunization schedule. The pneumococcal vaccine has only recently been introduced into routine use, and as pneumococcus is by far the most common cause of meningitis in children, we should see a significant reduction in the incidence of this dangerous infection in years to come. The bacteria listed in option (B) are the most common causes of meningitis in the neonate, and those listed in (C) are causes of otitis media. Although not listed, tuberculous meningitis is an indolent form of bacterial meningitis that must be suspected in a child who does not respond as expected to appropriate therapy.

22–A

Sensorineural hearing loss is the most common sequela of meningitis in children, occurring in as many as 30% of patients with pneumococcal meningitis. Severe neurodevelopmental disability (e.g., seizures, mental retardation) occurs in 10% to 20% of patients, and 50% have some sort of neurobehavioral morbidity, which may include subtle changes such as language delay and behavioral issues. Steroids, administered concomitantly with antibiotics in the acute phase, have been shown to reduce hearing loss in children with *H. influenzae* meningitis, and are used as an adjunct to therapy in some centers.

23–C

Low glucose (<75% of serum glucose) in the CSF is a sign of bacterial meningitis. It is caused by reduced glucose transport by inflamed cerebral tissue. Other signs in CSF include numerous white blood cells, typically with a neutrophil predominance, and elevated protein and microorganisms on gram stain. Numerous red cells may indicate a traumatic tap or, more rarely, a subarachnoid bleed, and are also associated with certain forms of aseptic meningitis.

24–C

Enterovirus is the primary cause of aseptic meningitis. Other viruses, including HSV, VZV, mumps, EBV, and arboviruses, can all infect the central nervous system (CNS) and cause meningitis or encephalitis. Cryptococcal meningitis is uncommon in immunocompetent children, but can occur in those with HIV, malignancy, or other forms of immunosuppression. The long-term prognosis of aseptic meningitis depends on the cause of the infection and the health of the child, but is generally more favorable than that of bacterial meningitis. Acute complications such as increased intracranial pressure and seizures occur in about 10% of children with enteroviral disease. As with bacterial meningitis, audiologic and neurodevelopmental evaluation should be part of routine follow-up examinations.

25–B, 26–D, 27–B, 28–E

For croup, the disease process involves obstruction and edema of the upper airways. Although the majority of patients are younger children, croup also can affect adolescents and even adults! The majority of patients never become symptomatic enough to prompt medical attention. For the patient in respiratory distress who has not responded to cool air mist or humidity, racemic epinephrine should be administered. Its effect primarily lies in stimulation of alpha-adrenergic receptors and a decrease in laryngeal mucosal edema. A child who responds to this treatment can safely be discharged from care after careful observation and an examination that reveals no stridor at rest, no color changes, and adequate air entry. Corticosteroids are often used to augment the anti-inflammatory process. Nebulized albuterol has not been shown to be effective in the management of croup. Wheezing after cool mist therapy may be found in the child whose croup involves the larger airways, but it is uncommon in children with croup. The most likely pathogens associated with croup are parainfluenza viruses, followed by influenza viruses, RSV, and adenoviruses.

Suspicion of epiglottitis warrants emergent, careful, and controlled examination of the airway. In the ill-appearing child with imminent upper airway obstruction, this should be done most preferably in the operating room with airway support readily available. Epiglottitis traditionally is caused by *H. influenzae* type B, but streptococcal species have also been implicated. The onset of symptoms in epiglottitis is generally much quicker than croup, and can result in obstruction of the airway within several hours. The advent of routine vaccination has helped decrease the incidence over the last 5 years. Antibiotics are indicated for the child who presents with a suspicion of epiglottitis or another suspected bacterial process (pneumonia, abscess); a clinical examination should support the diagnosis.

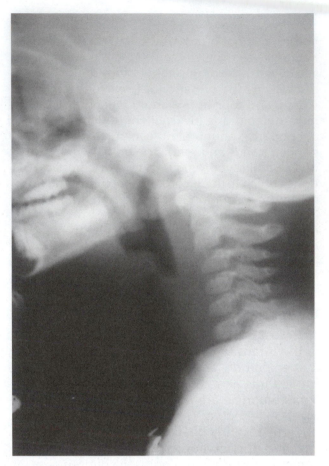

FIGURE A28-2 Epiglottitis in a 4-year-old child, with massive edema of the epiglottis, thickened aryepiglottic folds, and effacement of the valleculae. Used with permission from Marino B, Snead K, McMillan J. Blueprints in Pediatrics, 2nd ed. Malden: Blackwell Science, Inc., 2001: 158.

29–E

Blood-tinged sputum is usually a later finding. All of the other mentioned symptoms are generally earlier indications of a lodged foreign body in the trachea and mainstem bronchus.

30–A

It is also important to be aware of foreign body aspiration in the developmentally delayed patient at any age.

31–C

For a complete obstruction, the affected side will have a unilateral atelectasis with a shift of the heart to the affected side. In contrast, a partial obstruction allows a "ball-valve" mechanism for air-trapping on the affected side and a shift of the mediastinal structures away from the affected side.

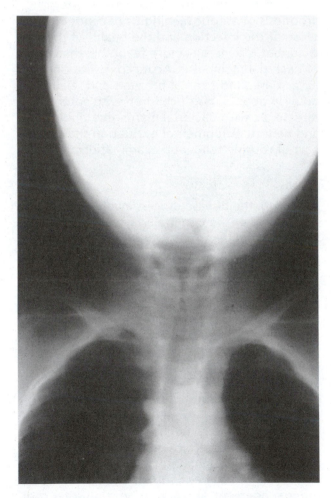

FIGURE A28-1 Croup in a 3-year-old child. Note the "steeple sign" indicative of subglottic narrowing. Used with permission from Marino B, Snead K, McMillan J. Blueprints in Pediatrics, 2nd ed. Malden: Blackwell Science, Inc., 2001: 157.

32–A

Aspiration of foreign bodies into the lower airway is much more common than tracheal obstruction.

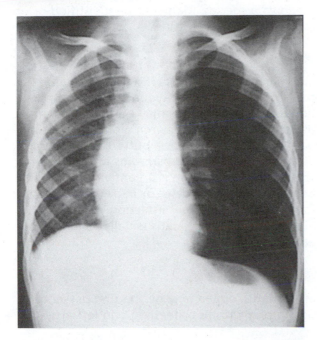

FIGURE A32 Expiratory film in foreign body aspiration with partial obstruction. The obstructed left lung is hyperinflated, whereas the heart (and mediastinum) are shifted to the right. Used with permission from Marino B, Snead K, McMillan J. Blueprints in Pediatrics, 2nd ed. Malden: Blackwell Science, Inc., 2001: 10.

33–D, 34–E, 35–E, 36–E

Pneumonia remains an important diagnosis in pediatrics. History, physical examination, and the underlying cause all usually depend on the age at presentation. Several risk factors are associated with bacterial pneumonia.

In neonates, ages 0 to 1 month, presentation and cause all suggest treatment for Group B streptococci, *E. coli*, and *L. monocytogenes* (common pathogens of neonatal sepsis).

In infants age 1 to 3 months, the most common causes of pneumonia remain viral (RSV, adenovirus, influenza). Viral pneumonia is generally preceded by upper respiratory tract infection symptoms, and can also be accompanied by signs and symptoms of respiratory distress. Many infants will also have nonspecific constitutional symptoms such as fever, lethargy, poor feeding, irritability, and vomiting. The physical examination may not be especially revealing. Bacterial pneumonia (predominantly *S. pneumoniae*) must also be considered. *Chlamydia trachomatis* pneumonia may pre-

sent in this age group in infants born to infected mothers, and is usually associated with a conjunctivitis.

In older infants and toddlers, the presentation may be similar to the above. Symptoms of cough, tachypnea, and respiratory distress may suggest pneumonia. Chest pain and dyspnea are seen less often than in the older child. Auscultation may reveal crackles and decreased breath sounds. Lobar consolidation may often cause diaphragmatic irritation, ileus, and a clinical picture consistent with an intra-abdominal process (as was true in the above case!). Viral agents remain prominent, but common bacterial pathogens now include *S. pneumoniae* (most common) and *H. influenzae* type B.

In older children, fever, chills, productive cough, dyspnea, and pleuritic chest pain may all be suggestive of pneumonia. Bacterial infections tend to increase with age in the hospitalized patient. Auscultative findings include crackles, dullness to percussion, and decreased breath sounds. Atypical pathogens such as *Mycoplasma pneumoniae* and *Chlamydia pneumoniae* are also included.

Chest x-ray may help define the pattern of involvement (lobar consolidation is often suggestive of bacterial pneumonia) and denote other processes involved (i.e., pleural effusions). CBC and blood culture (nearly 20% may have associated bacteremia) may provide aid in diagnosis and treatment. Inpatient treatment is warranted for respiratory distress and persistent hypoxia. Viral infections are generally self-limited and require supportive care. Bacterial pathogens require appropriate antibiotic coverage. Outpatient management with amoxicillin is appropriate for most cases of bacterial pneumonia. For cases of suspected *H. influenzae* or *S. aureus*, amoxicillin-clavulanic acid or a second- or third-generation cephalosporin may be required. For suspected mycoplasma pneumonia cases, erythromycin is the drug of choice. For inpatient therapy, where parenteral antibiotics may be required, cefuroxime or penicillin are appropriate choices for empiric therapy.

37–E

The immediate therapy for a child suffering from an acute asthma attack involves relief of acute airway constriction (via bronchodilators and oxygen therapy) and control of airway inflammation (via corticosteroids). Corticosteroids generally require 4 to 6 hours for effectiveness, but are indicated for initial therapy.

ANSWERS

38–D, 39–B

Asthma is characterized by a reversible component. The bronchoconstriction may result from a spectrum of different triggers. In an acute asthma attack, a low $PaCO_2$ indicates an adequate value secondary to tachypnea. (In fact, a "normal" $PaCO_2$ should immediately raise concern for inadequate ventilation and the patient rapidly tiring!) Physical findings of decreased breath sounds and no wheezing warrant concern over increasing obstruction. Other medications such as subcutaneous epinephrine or terbutaline can help decrease airway reactivity. Unfortunately, mortality has increased in recent years.

40–E

Previous RSV infection and poverty are also among the many risk factors for asthma.

41–D

Although anaphylaxis can evolve slowly or rapidly, the most common presentations occur within hours after exposure to an allergen. The reaction is primarily an IgE- and histamine-mediated reaction.

42–C, 43–A

Urticaria typically describes blanching, edematous, red and white evanescent plaques, which appear as hives on the skin or mucous membranes. They are pruritic, may be raised, and generally resolve within 24 hours. Angioedema is a similar process, involving swelling in a well-demarcated area devoid of pruritus. It is confined to the lower dermis and subcutaneous areas and also resolves within a few hours to days. Clinically, angioedema must be differentiated from cellulitis, erysipelas, lymphedema, and acute contact dermatitis. Angioedema that is associated with pruritus is also associated with urticaria, whereas angioedema due to C1 esterase deficiency is not usually pruritic.

44–E

The immediate concerns for these patients include support of the ABCs (airway, breathing, and circulation). Oxygen, epinephrine, and diphenhydramine may help alleviate reactive symptoms. Intubation may be warranted in cases of severe obstruction. Intravenous fluids are also indicated for intravascular volume support. Corticosteroids are indicated to help curb the inflammatory response and treat persistent symptoms.

45–E

Although RSV is the most important cause of bronchiolitis, it should be noted that there are several other causes, including *Mycoplasma* and *Chlamydia* species. Many can be identified using rapid viral antigen testing.

46–B

The majority of patients who are hospitalized require no more than oxygen and fluid support; however, some patients may benefit from added therapies. Although they remain controversial, bronchodilators (such as albuterol and racemic epinephrine) and corticosteroids may provide some benefit. Ribavirin is an antiviral that has been used in severe cases or in patients with risk factors. Although super-infection with pneumonia can occur, bronchiolitis usually requires no antibiotic therapy.

47–C

In neonates, apnea may be the first presenting sign, along with poor feeding and lethargy.

48–B

Palivizumab (Synagis) is an intramuscular injectable monoclonal antibody that provides passive prophylaxis against RSV. An RSV polyclonal antibody called RespiGam is also available, and both may be recommended for infants at risk during the winter months.

49–B

Cystic fibrosis is acquired through autosomal recessive inheritance and generally involves mutations of the CFTR gene located on the long arm of chromosome 7. It should be noted that genetic testing is available for the 14 most common mutations of this gene, which account for nearly 85% of cases.

50–C

CF may result in multisystemic complications. Respiratory complications remain the major contributors to morbidity and mortality. Progressive hypoxia and obstructive airway disease can also lead to chronic pulmonary hypertension and right heart failure. Gastrointestinal and endocrine complications are also numerous. Impaired male infertility is virtually universal. Pancreatic cancer is generally not a complication of CF.

51–D

Meconium ileus is virtually pathognomonic for CF in the newborn. Nearly 20% of patients present in this fashion. Clubbing, while almost always present in the CF patient, is usually not present in the neonate.

52–C

Pancreatic enzyme replacement along with nutritional support and vitamin supplementation (A, D, E, K) may help the CF patient to achieve near normal growth. Pulmonary therapies are multifaceted and include bronchodilators, anti-inflammatory agents, chest physiotherapy, as well as DNAse. Bacterial infections often exacerbate disease and should be treated with aminoglycosides in conjunction with other agents. Lung transplantation has become a viable option for those with poor pulmonary status and 1- to 2-year life expectancy.

53–D

Hyperbilirubinemia is of concern to the physician for two reasons. The first is the risk for neurotoxicity (kernicterus), which occurs when unconjugated bilirubin, normally tightly bound to albumin, reaches levels high enough to exceed the binding capacity of albumin and subsequently crosses the blood-brain barrier to damage cells of the brain. In full-term newborns this can occur at levels higher than 25–30 mg/dL. It occurs at lower levels in premature neonates. Although truly a pathologic diagnosis, signs of kernicterus include poor feeding, hypotonia, irritability, and seizures. Phototherapy and other methods of facilitating the excretion of bilirubin are effective at preventing kernicterus. Exchange transfusion, which directly removes bilirubin from the bloodstream, is used for dangerously high bilirubin levels (usually >25 mg/dL in full-term neonates), or in patients who fail to respond to phototherapy. The second reason for concern is that elevated bilirubin levels may indicate the other processes or disorders mentioned above, which should be identified and treated early. The management of the jaundiced newborn should be aimed both at preventing kernicterus and at identifying and treating the cause of the jaundice.

54–A

Most newborns will develop a transient unconjugated hyperbilirubinemia after birth, termed "physiologic jaundice." This type of jaundice begins *after* 24 hours of life, peaks at a level of 12–15 mg/dL of indirect (unconjugated) bilirubin at around 3 days of life, and returns to normal by 1 week of age. Hyperbilirubinemia that develops in the first 24 hours, increases at a rate greater than 5 mg/dL/day, includes a direct fraction of >2 mg/dL or 15% of total bilirubin, or lasts more than 1 week should be evaluated. Risk factors for the development of more severe physiologic jaundice include prematurity, maternal diabetes, breastfeeding and Asian or Native American ancestry.

55–B

Breastfeeding is *not* a cause of conjugated (direct) hyperbilirubinemia; it is caused by factors that slow or impede the excretion of bilirubin from the liver. These factors include 1) cholestasis due to paucity of bile ducts, neonatal hepatitis, TORCH infections, total parenteral nutrition, drugs, or neoplasms; 2) extrahepatic obstruction due to biliary atresia, common duct stenosis, cystic fibrosis, pancreatitis, orcholedochal cyst; and 3) genetic and metabolic disorders, such as disorders of bilirubin metabolism (e.g., Dubin-Johnson syndrome, Rotor syndrome), disorders of carbohydrate, amino acid or lipid metabolism, chromosomal disorders (e.g., trisomy 21, trisomy 18), and metabolic liver disease (e.g., Wilson's disease, α_1-antitrypsin deficiency).

56–D

The majority of clinically significant hemolysis from ABO incompatibility occurs when the mother is type O+ and the infant is type A+ or B+. ABO hemolytic disease is caused by preformed maternal anti-A or anti-B antibodies that passively cross the placenta late in pregnancy, or during delivery, and attack A or B antigen on fetal RBCs. Due to a relatively small number of antigen sites on fetal red blood cells, the direct Coombs' test (which looks for antibody-coated fetal RBCs) may be negative or weakly positive even when hemolysis is present; an indirect Coombs' test (which looks for maternal anti-A or anti-B antibodies in the fetal serum) is more sensitive. Although 25% of pregnancies have the potential for ABO incompatibility, only around 10% of these develop hemolysis. Rh incompatibility is much rarer than ABO incompatibility, and causes a much more severe form of hemolytic disease. All women identified as Rh negative during pregnancy should have the infant's blood tested prenatally or immediately after delivery for ABO and Rh type, hemoglobin, total bilirubin, and direct Coombs' reactivity.

57–C

Pulmonary edema is *not* a hallmark finding on chest x-ray of RDS. The classic triad of radiological findings are low lung volume, air bronchograms, and a "ground-glass" appearance of the lung parenchyma. It is interesting to note that the chest x-ray can change significantly following a single dose of exogenous surfactant. In the case of an infant with respiratory distress, a very similar chest x-ray can also be the result of pneumonia due to Group B streptococcal sepsis, and therefore a rule-out sepsis workup including antibiotics must always be carried out.

58–B

Alveolar type II cells are responsible for the production and packaging of surfactant, which is stored in lamellar bodies within the cells prior to its release.

59–B

Hypoglycemia is *not* a complication of exogenous surfactant administration. The other complications listed occur as a result of instilling fluid into the air spaces and a rapid change in lung compliance.

60–C

Antenatal steroids have been associated with both a decrease in severity of RDS as well as a decrease in incidence of intracranial hemorrhage.

61–C

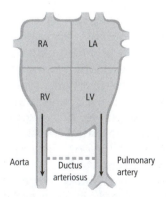

FIGURE A61 Transposition of the great vessels. Used with permission from Rudolf M, Levene M. Paediatrics and Child Health. Oxford: Blackwell Science, Ltd., 1999: 254.

TGA is associated with the classic "egg on a string" appearance of the heart. The "boot-shaped" heart indicates tetralogy of Fallot, the "snowman" appearance indicates TAPVR; and the "sail" sign describes the thymus associated with a pneumomediastinum.

62–B

The ECG findings in TGA are normal and can evolve into right axis deviation with right ventricular hypertrophy as the right ventricle continues to support systemic circulation.

63–C

Tetralogy of Fallot is *not* associated with an atrial septal defect.

64–C

Coarctation of the aorta is hallmarked by the finding of lower blood pressure in the lower extremities when compared to the upper extremities. This is because systemic blood flow is restricted by the stenotic aortic arch and is instead provided by right to left shunting of blood through a patent ductus arteriosus.

65–D

The definitive diagnosis of malrotation is an abnormally placed ligament of Treitz in the right upper instead of left upper quadrant, and a cecum in the left lower instead of right lower quadrant. Retroperitoneal attachment is inadequate and the mesenteric pedicle is narrow, which can easily lead to volvulus. The symptom of bilious vomiting indicates the presence of a complete or intermittent obstruction associated with a volvulus.

66–B

A malrotation with associated volvulus is a surgical emergency and a pediatric surgeon must be immediately consulted for surgical intervention. A barium enema to reconfirm abnormal placement of the cecum is unnecessary because the diagnosis is already confirmed.

67–C

Malrotation occurs when the small intestines abnormally rotate in utero, resulting in malposition in the abdomen and posterior fixation of the mesentery. When the intestine attaches improperly to the mesentery, it is at risk for twisting (volvulus) on its vascular supply, the superior mesenteric artery.

68–C

The metabolic derangement resulting from malrotation and volvulus is a severe metabolic acidosis due to bowel ischemia and infarction. This derangement should be corrected by aggressive therapy, including intubation with control of breathing and administration of fluids and alkali (NaHCO$_3$).

69–B

Atrioventricular nodal reentry tachycardia accounts for 90% of causes of SVT in children.

70–B

The combination of a short PR interval in conjunction with a delta wave comprises the Wolff-Parkinson-White (WPW) syndrome and indicates an abnormal retrograde conduction pathway between the ventricles and the atria. This condition is associated with an increased risk of serious arrhythmias, and can be treated with ablation of the abnormal conduction pathway.

71–D

Verapamil is contraindicated for use in infants with SVT because its vasodilating and negative inotropic effects may lead to hypotension and

cardiac arrest in these patients. Older children with SVT can be taught to do vagal maneuvers such as squatting to control their symptoms. Although recommended in adults, carotid massage is generally not performed in infants and children due to the risk of occluding cerebral blood flow. Stable patients can be treated with vagal maneuvers or medications such as adenosine or digoxin; cardioversion should be administered to patients with signs of hemodynamic instability as soon as possible.

72–D

In WPW syndrome, a bypass tract through a Kent bundle is present, whereby atrial conduction bypasses the atrioventricular node, entering an area of the left or right ventricle or septum directly.

73–B

21-Hydroxylase deficiency accounts for 90% of the cases of CAH. Deficiency of this enzyme leads to decreased production of mineralocorticoids and cortisol and an overproduction of androgens causing virilization of a female. It can also present as a salt-wasting deficiency in which symptoms of emesis, salt wasting, dehydration, and shock develop in the first 2 to 4 weeks of life. Male infants born with the defect have no genital abnormalities (Fig. A73).

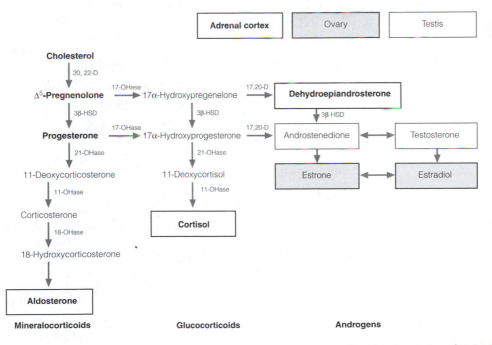

FIGURE A73 A schematic of steroidogenesis in the adrenal cortex. Used with permission from Marino B, Snead K, McMillan J. Blueprints in Pediatrics, 2nd ed. Malden: Blackwell Science, Inc., 2001: 73.

74–D

Measurement of elevated levels of 17-hydroxy-progesterone confirms the diagnosis of CAH. Interestingly, prenatal diagnosis in the siblings of children with 21-hydroxylase deficiency can be made by measuring elevated levels of 17-hydroxy-progesterone in amniotic fluid and HLA typing, because siblings who share the defect have the same HLA type.

75–A

Hypernatremia is associated with 11-hydroxylase deficiency, unlike the hyponatremic salt wasting that occurs with 21-hydroxylase deficiency (the patient in this case). 11-Hydroxylase deficiency is also associated with hypokalemia and hypertension.

76–D

Testosterone is *not* part of the therapy for 21-hydroxylase deficiency. Treatment includes cortisol, mineralocorticoids, surgical correction if necessary, and appropriate genetic counseling and recommendations for the family.

77–E

All of the symptoms mentioned are possible. Classically, fever, emesis, and periumbilical pain are followed by right lower quadrant pain (at McBurney's point), guarding, and the obturator/psoas signs. Perforation typically occurs 36 hours after pain begins, and may manifest with signs of peritoneal irritation.

78–E

These diagnoses make the diagnosis of appendicitis difficult, and highlight the importance of an adequate history and physical examination, and index of suspicion for these conditions.

79–D

The appendix typically tends to perforate 36 to 48 hours after pain begins. This can be quite common in the younger child and toddler, who may have a longer duration of symptoms before diagnosis. The retrocecal appendix usually does not induce right lower quadrant pain until after perforation occurs.

80–D

A typical presentation is quite common in children, particularly with retrocecal appendicitis.

The diagnosis is best made clinically, which includes a rectal examination to detect tenderness or masses. Appendicitis typically affects the child between 10 to 15, with less than 10% under age 5.

81–B

In DKA, metabolic acidosis occurs from ketone production and dehydration. The natural physiologic response to this is a compensatory respiratory alkalosis.

82–B

In states of acidosis, the inability of potassium to stay in the cell results in a hyperkalemia. Global catecholamine release in the face of a general lack of cellular glucose availability can result in symptoms of hypoglycemia. The catabolic mediators produce ketone bodies, which will manifest as ketonuria until the process is reversed. Inadequate insulin dosage can be a common trigger for DKA.

83–A

Type I diabetes mellitus has many proposed causes; genetic, autoimmune, and environmental factors have all been implicated. The basic disorder is characterized by a lack of insulin production at the cellular level. It is only after 90% of pancreatic B-cell function has been destroyed that loss of insulin secretion becomes clinically significant. The mainstays of medical management include insulin replacement therapy, diet and exercise modification, and proper daily monitoring of blood glucose levels. Long-term complications include microvascular disease and accelerated large vessel atherosclerosis.

84–D

Type II diabetes mellitus is becoming more of a concern, as an increasing number of cases are being found in the pediatric population. The primary underlying abnormality is thought to be due to insulin resistance. Most affected patients are overweight, and the presence of acanthosis nigricans (a hyperpigmentation with a velvety texture, often found on the nape of the neck or antecubital fossa) is commonly found on physical examination. Insulin may be required for some patients, but many patients can also be treated with oral medications. Nevertheless, diet and exercise remain the mainstays of any therapeutic regimen.

85–D

Testicular torsion most commonly occurs in the adolescent male and is a surgical emergency. Most patients lack the posterior mesenteric attachment to the tunica vaginalis that keeps the testis from rotating around the spermatic cord. In some cases the attachment may be too narrow. The "blue-dot" sign is associated with torsion of the appendix testis (an embryonic remnant of the developing gonad) and may be observed as a tender, discolored nodule on the upper pole of the testicle. Torsion of the appendix testis can be managed often with analgesics alone.

86–E

Varicocele is a dilation of the venous plexus of the spermatic cord and presents classically as a palpable mass ("bag of worms" appearance) above the left testis. Hydrocele is produced by accumulation of peritoneal fluid inside a patent processus vaginalis and can be associated with hernias. Inguinal hernias can also be a cause of scrotal swelling.

87–C

Mumps orchitis classically presents within 1 week following parotitis, although it may occur in the absence of salivary gland involvement. Immunization history should be obtained. These patients may have fever, pain, and swelling for 4 to 10 days. Occasionally, infection can result in testicular atrophy and decreased fertility.

88–C

Cryptorchidism is defined by testes that have not fully descended into the scrotum and cannot be manipulated into the scrotum with gentle pressure. It occurs in 3% to 4% of term males and is more common in premature babies. Testes that remain outside the scrotum are at increased risk for traumatic injury and malignancy. The majority of cases resolve by age 1 year. Surgical repair has a much higher success rate than hormonal therapy.

89–E

Generalized seizures are always associated with impaired consciousness and are indicative of bilateral hemispheric involvement. Tonic–clonic (sustained contraction followed by rhythmic contractions), absence (brief staring episodes signified by symmetric 3 per second spike and wave pattern on EEG), and atonic (abrupt total loss of muscle tone) are types of generalized seizure.

These seizures can also be followed by a post-ictal phase of confusion and lethargy. Infantile spasms are a type of generalized seizure that present between 2 to 8 months and are recurrent mixed flexor–extensor contractions that last 10 to 30 seconds each. They are frequently associated with developmental milestone loss and can also be associated with neurocutaneous disorders.

90–A

Only complex partial seizures are associated with impaired consciousness. Partial seizures involve foci in one hemisphere and can occasionally progress to generalized convulsions.

91–E

Status epilepticus is defined as prolonged or recurrent seizure activity (usually >20 to 30 minutes) with no return of consciousness. The ABCs should be evaluated and maintained. Benzodiazepines can initially break the seizure and can be followed by doses of phenytoin (or fosphenytoin) or phenobarbital (used in neonates and younger children). Assessing and treating underlying causes such as metabolic derangements, underlying infection, or trauma should be included in the management.

92–A

TABLE A92. Common Indications and Side Effects of Anticonvulsants		
MEDICATION	INDICATIONS	SIDE EFFECTS/TOXICITY
Carbamazepine (Tegretol)	Partial, tonic–clonic	Diplopia, nausea and vomiting, ataxia, leukopenia, thrombocytopenia
Ethosuximide (Zarontin)	Absence	Rash, anorexia, leukopenia, aplastic anemia
Phenobarbital (Luminal)	Tonic–clonic, partial	Hyperactivity, sedation, nystagmus, ataxia
Phenytoin (Dilantin)	Tonic–clonic, partial	Rash, nystagmus, ataxia, drug-induced lupus, gum hyperplasia, anemia, leukopenia, polyneuropathy
Valproic acid (Depakene, Depakote)	Tonic–clonic, absence, partial	Hepatotoxicity, nausea and vomiting, abdominal pain, weight loss, weight gain, anemia, leukopenia, thrombocytopenia

Used with permission from Marino B, Snead K, McMillan J. Blueprints in Pediatrics, 2nd ed. Malden: Blackwell Science, Inc., 2001: 234.

ANSWERS

Ethosuximide is generally used to treat absence seizures and is associated with rash, anorexia, and blood dyscrasias. Treatment with anti-epileptic medications requires knowledge of their uses and toxicity. Monitoring drug levels and noting their interactions can help in management.

93–D

A variety of extraintestinal manifestations may either precede or accompany GI symptoms. Additional findings may include pyoderma gangrenosum, hepatobiliary findings, sacroiliitis, nephrolithiasis, and thromboembolic disease. Approximately one-third of patients have at least one of these manifestations. Acanthosis nigricans is a skin finding commonly found with type II diabetes.

94–A

Crohn's disease extends transmurally whereas ulcerative colitis is limited to the mucosal surface.

95–E

Goals of therapy include control of inflammation, providing adequate nutrition and growth support, and encouraging the patient/family to lead a normal life. Aminosalicylates such as sulfasalazine are indicated for colonic disease. Corticosteroids are useful for small intestinal disease, and also in conjunction with other aminosalicylates. Surgery may be helpful and warranted in many IBD patients. Metoclopramide generally has no role in IBD management.

96–C

Many patients with Crohn disease present insidiously and have only a right lower quadrant fullness or mass on initial examination. Delayed growth and sexual development and nutrient losses may precede the initial manifestations. When Crohn disease affects the large intestine, it is clinically hard to distinguish from ulcerative colitis, as they both present with bloody diarrhea, abdominal pain, and urgency. Bleeding, toxic megacolon, and abscesses can be complications of ulcerative colitis. Internal/external fistula formation are the most common complications of Crohn disease, and occurs in up to 40% of patients.

TABLE A96. Comparison of Crohn Disease and Ulcerative Colitis

FEATURE	CROHN DISEASE	ULCERATIVE COLITIS
Malaise, fever, weight loss	Common	Common
Rectal bleeding	Sometimes	Usual
Abdominal mass	Common	Rare
Abdominal pain	Common	Common
Perianal disease	Common	Rare
Ileal involvement	Common	None (backwash ileitis)
Strictures	Common	Unusual
Fistula	Common	Unusual
Skip lesions	Common	Not present
Transmural involvement	Usual	Not present
Crypt abscesses	Unusual	Usual
Granulomas	Common	Not present
Risk of cancer	Slightly increased	Greatly increased

Modified from Andreoli TE, Carpenter CJ, Plum F, et al. Cecil Essentials of Medicine. Philadelphia: WB Saunders, 1986: 746.

97–D

Hypotension is the last of the listed clinical manifestations of dehydration to appear. Tachycardia is often the first in children, although it is very nonspecific.

98–C

This patient is moderately dehydrated based on the following parameters: 5% to 10% weight loss; dry mucous membranes; altered mental status; absent tears; sunken eyes; oliguria; urine specific gravity 1.025; elevated BUN; and pH between 7.30 and 6.92.

TABLE A98. Clinical Features in Estimating the Severity of Dehydration

CLINICAL FEATURE	MILD	MODERATE	SEVERE
Mucosa of mouth	Dry	Dry	Dry
Reported urine output	Normal (at least × 3 in 24 hours)	Reduced in last 24 hours	No urine in last 12 hours
Mental state	Normal	Lethargic or stuporous	Irritable
Pulse	Normal	Tachycardic	Tachycardic
Blood pressure	Normal	Normal	Low
Capillary refilling	Normal	Slow	Very slow
Fontanelle	Normal	Sunken	Very sunken
Skin and eye turgor	Normal	Reduced	Very reduced
Percentage dehydrated	<5%	5–10%	>10%

Used with permission from Rudolf M, Levene M. Paediatrics and Child Health. Oxford: Blackwell Science, Ltd., 1999: 117.

99–C

This patient has isotonic dehydration given her serum sodium of 135 mEq/L. Isotonic dehydration is the most common form of dehydration and suggests that either compensation has occurred or water losses are equal to salt losses. Hypotonic dehydration in children is caused by electrolyte loss in stools, or can also occur in children supplemented with free water or dilute juices. Hypertonic dehydration is uncommon in children.

100–C

Brain edema due to excessive fluid shifts is a complication of rapid fluid correction in less than 48 hours for hypertonic (hypernatremic) dehydration. Brain swelling occurs as a result of rapid entry of free water into neuronal cells with high sodium concentrations. Brain edema may lead to increased intracranial pressure with mental status changes or hypoventilation and bradycardia.

101–C

The most common agent to cause acute gastroenteritis is rotavirus. *Staphylococcus aureus* and *Clostridium perfringens* are associated with food poisoning. *E. coli* frequently causes infectious diarrhea, especially watery traveler's diarrhea. Adenovirus is generally associated with respiratory illness, although extension of viral inflammation into the GI tract could also cause gastric irritation and symptoms of gastroenteritis.

102–E

Outpatient oral rehydration is the treatment of choice for patients with mild dehydration who are able to tolerate food or fluids orally. Inpatient IV administration of fluids is indicated only if oral rehydration is not possible.

103–B

Giardia lamblia is the most common cause of parasitic watery diarrhea in the United States.

104–C

Clostridium difficile toxin is often associated with a history of antibiotic overuse. *Salmonella*, *Shigella*, enterohemorrhagic *E. coli*, and *Yersinia enterocolitica* may be associated with blood, mucus, and fecal leukocytes.

105–B

Visible gastric peristaltic waves are often seen with pyloric stenosis. Simian crease is associated with trisomy-21 (Down syndrome), which can also have duodenal atresia and thus have the radiographic finding of a "double-bubble" sign. Bloody stools are not common in pyloric stenosis.

106–A

Inguinal hernia is the most common condition requiring surgical correction in term newborns. Pyloric stenosis is the second most common.

107–D

The surgical treatment for pyloric stenosis is pyloromyotomy, which involves making a longitudinal incision through the external pyloric musculature and suturing it in a lateral direction (at 90 degrees from the original).

108–D

The metabolic derangement resulting from pyloric stenosis is hypokalemic metabolic alkalosis. The loss of gastric secretions through emesis requires replacement of KCl and alkali before surgical correction can be performed.

109–D, 110–C, 111–C, 112–C

Intestinal lead points include the given answers, and more rarely Henoch-Schönlein purpura, fecaliths, traumatic hematoma, and cystic fibrosis. A duodenal ulcer is not generally a likely lead point.

The physical findings can range from peritoneal signs to a normal examination. In a majority of patients (up to 80%) a sausage-shaped mass is palpable in the right side of the abdomen. Hepatosplenomegaly is generally not seen.

In the overwhelming majority of patients, a cause is not found (up to 90%). The peak age of occurrence is between 3 to 18 months, and a specific lead point should be sought in older children. Pneumatic and/or hydrostatic enema can be both diagnostic and therapeutic. These methods are successful in the majority of patients, but are also accompanied by a recurrence rate of nearly 15%. Open surgical reduction may be required. Supportive care with fluids and nasogastric decompression is the mainstay of initial management.

The differential diagnosis for intussusception should include those entities that are commonly associated with acute abdominal pain. This list is quite extensive, but generally does not include food allergies, which typically present with chronic abdominal symptoms.

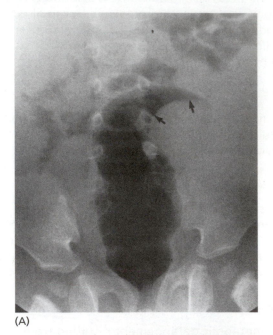

(A)

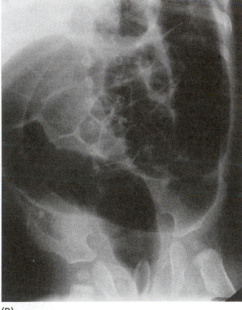

(B)

FIGURE A112 Air enema of a child with intussusception. **(A)** The intussusception is clearly demarcated indenting the colonic lumen (see arrows). **(B)** Following reduction, air is now seen in the small bowel. Used with permission from Rudolf M, Levene M. Paediatrics and Child Health. Oxford: Blackwell Science, Ltd., 1999: 136.

113–A

Peptic ulcer disease is an upper GI source of blood, and therefore presents with melena or heme-positive stool, not rectal bleeding. Blood is chemically

changed during transit through the gut to appear dark or tarry. Very rarely, however, a briskly bleeding duodenal ulcer may appear as rectal bleeding due to rapid transit time through the intestine.

114–D

All of the procedures listed should be performed to stabilize a patient with an active upper GI bleed. Gastric lavage should be performed with warm saline (not ice cold, as this can cause hypothermia and inhibit clotting) and should be repeated until the bleeding is controlled. In addition to the above measures, intravenous H_2 blockers should be administered to reduce gastric acidity. Endoscopy is usually performed once the patient is stable to determine the source of the bleeding.

115–C

Meckel's diverticulum, the most common anomaly of the GI tract, is usually composed of heterotopic gastric tissue. The most common presentation is painless rectal bleeding. Meckel's diverticulum is typically located in the small intestine within 2 feet of the ileocecal valve, has a peak incidence of bleeding at 2 years of age, and is present in 2% of the population (the "2–2-2" rule). The diagnosis is made by performing a special nuclear scan, called a Meckel's scan, to identify the ectopic acid-secreting cells in the diverticulum.

116–D

The differential for GI bleeds in children varies based on the age of the patient. For example, in the neonate, swallowed maternal blood and milk allergy are common causes of lower GI bleeds, whereas IBD and hemorrhoids are likely causes in the adolescent patient. Lower GI bleeds are more common than upper GI bleeds, and rectal bleeding is the most common presentation. Melena usually suggests an upper GI bleed, but the appearance of melena can also be caused by ingestion of iron, bismuth, blackberries, or spinach.

117–C

Antibiotics are *not* indicated in the conservative management of toxic synovitis.

118–B

The patient has septic arthritis and needs immediate surgical intervention involving open joint drainage to preserve the limb. A dose of IV antibiotics with good *S. aureus* coverage, such as nafcillin, should also be started immediately. A bone scan would not give additional information at this point because the definitive diagnosis has already been established by the purulent joint fluid.

119–C

Even in patients with sickle cell disease who have asplenia, the most common organism causing septic arthritis is still *S. aureus.* These patients also have increased risk of acquiring infections due to encapsulated organisms such as *Salmonella typhi.*

120–E

Gonoccocal arthritis associated with disseminated gonococcal infection is the most common cause of polyarthritis or monoarticular arthritis in adolescents.

121–D

The diagnosis of SLE is based on clinical evaluation and requires 4 of the 11 criteria for 96% certainty of disease.

122–C

Polyarteritis nodosa, a vasculitic syndrome, is *not* a sequelae of JRA. Uveitis tends to be acute, with decreased visual acuity and erythema; patients may also develop ankylosing spondylitis and features of Reiter syndrome.

123–D

An 80% of all children with JRA will "outgrow" their disease and the prognosis is more favorable in young females with pauciarticular disease. It is, however, less favorable in the child with seropositive polyarticular disease.

124–D

X-ray changes in JRA are usually minimal. Morning stiffness does occur even in children and can be alleviated with early rising, warm morning baths, and heating pads and electric blankets. Pain symptoms are variable with some children having no pain and others with significant discomfort. Growth retardation occurs especially if steroids have been used to treat JRA. Some catch-up growth does occur during periods of remission.

125–D

Nursemaid's elbows are usually easily treated in the clinic setting. Pressure over the radial head as the arm is flexed and supinated will correct the subluxed radial head. There is often no need for x-ray if there is a strong history of the patient's arm being pulled and no tenderness to palpation of the bones of the wrist and arm. If there is doubt about the presence of a fracture, an x-ray should be obtained before trying to reduce the elbow in the clinic or emergency room. After reduction, there is almost immediate resolution of pain and recovery of normal range of motion.

126–E

Interestingly, patients are often able to lightly flex or extend at the elbow but always hold arm in pronation until corrected. After reduction the arm should not be splinted, because this slows recovery, and ice, ibuprofen, or acetaminophen can be recommended for pain and swelling.

127–A

No additional treatment beyond manual repositioning of the subluxed radial head as described is necessary. Although the problem may recur, it resolves with maturation.

128–C

Dislocation of the shoulder is uncommon in childhood and becomes more frequent in adolescents. The younger a child is at the time of initial dislocation, the higher the chance of developing a recurrent dislocation. Because of the high recurrence of dislocation, some orthopedic surgeons favor early reconstruction rather than conservative watchful management.

129–C

Splenic ultrasound is *not* helpful in establishing the diagnosis of sickle cell disease. Rather, it would only be useful to identify splenic enlargement and not the cause.

130–B

Sickle cell trait is generally an asymptomatic condition in which an individual may rarely exhibit painless hematuria and/or an inability to concentrate the urine. The importance of diagnosing sickle cell trait is to provide proper genetic counseling for those individuals who wish to have children. Answer (A) represents homozygous sickle cell disease (the patient in this case). Answer (C) is hemoglobin sickle cell disease, and answer (D) is for an individual without hemoglobinopathy.

ANSWERS

131–C

The substitution of a valine for glutamine in the sixth position of the β-globin chain is the hallmark of sickle cell disease.

132–D

Splenic autoinfarction is caused by microvascular obstruction as sickled cells pass through the spleen. The associated infarction and fibrosis of splenic tissue leads to a gradual regression in splenic size, usually by age 4 years. The diminished capability of the spleen to filter encapsulated organisms places the infant and child at great risk for overwhelming sepsis, meningitis, pneumonia, arthritis, and osteomyelitis.

133–D

The diagnosis of SCFE in a patient should be treated by immediate surgical consultation. Casting or splinting is not effective, and prolonged disunion of the bones can lead to permanent damage.

134–A

Trauma is *not* a contributing factor to SCFE. Associated factors include obesity, male predominance, African American race, and certain endocrine disorders such as hypothyroidism.

135–A

The primary goal of treatment is prevention of further misalignment.

136–B

Avascular necrosis and late degenerative changes similar to those seen with osteoarthritis may occur as long-term consequences of SCFE.

137–B

Upper motor neuron lesions are usually associated with "upward" direction Babinski reflex of toes. Guillain-Barré syndrome is a progressive demyelination of the peripheral nervous system (lower motor neurons), and therefore produces a pattern of ascending weakness with absent DTRs, normal Babinski reflex (downward), and intact sensation.

138–D

Stool cultures obtained from patients with Guillain-Barré syndrome at the onset of weakness are positive for *C. jejuni* in more than 25% of cases. Although in most cases the cause is unknown, a recent history of viral infection is often obtained from patients.

139–B

The onset of classic Guillain-Barré progression occurs in an ascending pattern and is followed by recovery in an opposite direction (descending) pattern. A variant of Guillain-Barré syndrome known as Miller-Fisher syndrome starts with acute external ophthalmoplegia, and progresses in a descending pattern. Although recovery is usually complete, the primary morbidity from group B streptococci is respiratory failure, sometimes requiring intubation.

140–A

Blurry vision is *not* associated with Guillain-Barré syndrome.

141–A

Lead poisoning is a major preventive health issue in primary care pediatrics. Exposure to lead based paint is the main cause, and a blood lead level above 20 defines lead poisoning. Developmental delay can be one of the associated findings that may include cognitive and neurologic impairment. Pica refers to a propensity to put nonedible objects in the mouth, and is commonly associated with the intake of flaking lead paint. Anorexia, nausea, vomiting, abdominal pain, and constipation can occur. For severe cases, seizures, encephalopathy, and coma may result. Lead poisoning (along with iron deficiency and thalassemia) commonly is associated with a microcytic anemia. The CDC recommends universal screening for lead poisoning at 12 months and 2 years of age.

142–C

Of the four domains of development, language is the best indicator for future intellectual achievement.

143–B

Cerebral palsy is a disorder of motor movements and posture, resulting from an insult to the motor area of the brain. Injuries may occur before, during, or after birth. Although most patients have perinatal complications resulting in cerebral palsy, many cases have no known cause. Abnormal posture, visual/oral function, posture, tone, and primitive/muscle-stretch reflexes are usually present and are static rather than progressive in nature. Regressing motor skills usually suggests a different subset of diagnoses. Mental retardation and intellectual impairment may be present in nearly half of cases, but is not always present. A multidisciplinary approach to care best serves these patients and their families.

144—C, B, D, A

The sequence for sexual development in females is thelarche (breast buds), height growth spurt, pubic hair, and menarche. The events of puberty in both sexes occur in predictable sequences but may vary in their timing and velocity for each individual.

TABLE A144-1. Normal Developmental Milestones

AGE	GROSS MOTOR	VISUAL/FINE MOTOR	LANGUAGE	SOCIAL
1 month	Raises head slightly from prone, makes crawling movements	Tight grasp, visually fixes/follows to midline	Alerts to sound	Regards face
2 months	Head held in midline, lifts chest off table *3 months:* Holds head steadily, supports on forearms in prone	Follows past midline, fist no longer clenched *3 months:* Hands open at rest, responds to visual threat	Social smile *3 months:* Coos	Parent recognition *3 months:* Reaches for familiar objects/people
4 months	Rolls front to back, supports on wrists *5 months:* Rolls back to front, sits with support	Brings hands to midline, reaches with arms in unison, grabs rattle	Laughs, orients to voice, needs expressed through differential cry *5 months:* orients to bell (localizes laterally)	Enjoys looking around environment
6 months	Sits unsupported, puts feet in mouth when supine *7 months:* Creeps	Reaches with either hand, object transfer, uses raking grasp	Babbles, imitates sound *7 months:* orients to bell (localized indirectly)	Recognizes strangers; expresses displeasure when toy or parent removed
8 months	Comes to sit *9 months:* Crawls, pulls to stand	Object inspection *9 months:* pincer grasp, holds bottle, probes with forefinger	"Dada" (indiscriminate) *9 months:* waves bye-bye, "Mama" (indiscriminate), understands "no"	Fingerfeeding *9 months:* Explores environment, plays pat-a-cake
10 months	Cruises, walks when led with both hands *11 months:* Walks when led with one hand	—	"Dada/Mama" (discriminate), orients to bell (directly) *11 months:* Follows 1-step command with gesture	—
12 months	Walks alone	Mature pincer grasp, marks paper with pencil, voluntary release	2 words other than "Dada/Mama," immature jargon *13 months:* Uses 3 words *14 months:* Follows 1-step command without gesture	Imitates actions, comes when called, cooperates with dressing
15 months	Creeps up stairs, walks backward	Scribbles with crayons (imitation), stacks 2 blocks (imitation), uses spoon and cup	Uses 4 to 6 words *17 months:* 7 to 20 words, points to 5 body parts, mature jargon	Give/takes toys, tests limits and rules, plays games with parents

ANSWERS

TABLE A144-1. (Continued)

AGE	GROSS MOTOR	VISUAL/FINE MOTOR	LANGUAGE	SOCIAL
18 months	Runs, throws toy from standing	Spontaneous scribble, feeds self, turns 2–3 pages at a time, stacks 3 blocks	2-word combinations *19 months:* Knows 8 body parts	Copies parent in tasks, likes to play with other children
21 months	Squats in play, goes up steps	Stacks 5 blocks	2-word sentences, uses 50 words	Asks to have food, go to toilet
24 months	Up/down steps without help, throws ball overhand	Stacks 7 blocks, turns pages one at a time, imitates pencil stroke, removes pants and shoes	Uses pronouns inappropriately, follows 2-step commands	Listens to short stories, parallel play
30 months	Jumps with both feet off floor	Holds pencil in adult fashion, horizontal and vertical strokes, unbuttons	Uses pronouns appropriately, concept of "1," repeats 2-digit forward	Tells first and last name, gets self drink without help
3 years	Rides tricycle, goes up steps with alternate feet, kicks ball	Copies circle, undresses completely, dresses partially, stacks 8 blocks	Uses 250 words, 3-word sentences, understands concept of "2," plural/past tense, speech 75% intelligible	Group play, takes turns, knows full name/age/sex, shares toys
4 years	Hops, alternates feet going down stairs	Copies cross, buttons clothing, dresses completely, catches ball *4.5 years:* Copies square	Asks questions, knows colors, song, or poem from memory	Tells "tall tales," cooperative play with a group of children
5 years	Skips alternating feet, balances on one foot	Copies triangle, ties shoes, spreads with knife	Prints first name, asks word meanings, tells simple story	Competitive games, helps in household tasks, abides by rules

TABLE A144-2. Tanner Staging of Secondary Sex Characteristics

BREAST DEVELOPMENT

Stage 1 Preadolescent; elevation of papilla only.
Stage 2 Breast bud; elevation of breast and papilla as small mound; enlargement of areolar diameter (11.15 ± 1.10).
Stage 3 Further enlargement and elevation of breast and areola; no separation of their contours (12.15 ± 1.09).
Stage 4 Projection of areola and papilla to form secondary mound above level of breast (13.11 ± 1.15).
Stage 5 Mature stage; projection of papilla only due to recession of areola to general contour of breast (15.33 ± 1.74).
Note: Stages 4 and 5 may not be distinct in some patients.

GENITAL DEVELOPMENT (MALE)

Stage 1 Preadolescent; testes, scrotum, and penis about same size and proportion as in early childhood.
Stage 2 Enlargement of scrotum and testes, skin of scrotum reddens and changes in texture; little or no enlargement of penis (11.64 ± 1.07).
Stage 3 Enlargement of penis, first mainly in length; further growth of testes and scrotum (12.85 ± 1.04).
Stage 4 Increased size of penis with growth in breadth and development of glans; further enlargement of testes and scrotum and increased darkening of scrotal skin (13.77 ± 1.02).
Stage 5 Genitalia adult in size and shape (14.92 ± 1.10).

PUBIC HAIR (MALE AND FEMALE)

Stage 1 Preadolescent; vellus over pubes no further developed than that over abdominal wall (i.e., no pubic hair).
Stage 2 Sparse growth of long, slightly pigmented downy hair, straight or only slightly curled, chiefly at base of penis or along labia. (Male: 13.44 ± 1.09. Female: 11.69 ± 1.21.)
Stage 3 Considerably darker, coarser, and more curled; hair spreads sparsely over junction of pubes. (Male: 13.9 ± 1.04. Female 12.36 ± 1.10.)
Stage 4 Hair resembles adult in type; distribution still considerably smaller than in adult. No spread to medial surface of thighs. (Male: 14.36 ± 1.08. Female: 12.95 ± 1.06.)
Stage 5 Adult in quantity and type with distribution of the horizontal pattern. (Male: 15.18 ± 1.07. Female: 14.41 ± 1.12.)
Stage 6 Spread up linea alba: "male escutcheon."

Used with permission from Marino B, Snead K, McMillan J. Blueprints in Pediatrics, 2nd ed. Malden: Blackwell Science, Inc., 2001: 52.

145–D

The management of acute PSGN is mainly supportive, as it is usually a self-limited disorder. Over 98% of children with PSGN make a full recovery, although the symptoms may take months to resolve. Complications such as hypertension and edema are treated with vasodilators, diuretics, and fluid restriction. If the patient has a positive streptococcal culture of skin or throat at the time of diagnosis, appropriate antibiotic therapy should be initiated. Steroids and other immunosuppressants have not been shown to affect course or outcome. The prognosis for other types of glomerulonephritis is much less favorable. For example, most boys and 20% of girls with Alport syndrome will progress to end-stage renal disease (ESRD) by mid-adulthood; those with rapidly progressive glomerulonephritis (a rare and devastating form of GN) usually become dialysis dependent within a few years.

146–C

Increased urine output is not associated with renal failure. Decreased urine output (oliguria, defined as urine output less than 0.5 mL/kg per hour in infants, or 500 mL/1.73 m^2 per day in older children) or absence of urine output (anuria) are signs of renal failure. Diminished renal function is accompanied by azotemia (accumulation of nitrogen waste products), electrolyte imbalance (particularly hyperkalemia), and fluid retention. Hypertension, anemia, and metabolic acidosis may also occur. Most cases of acute renal failure in children are prerenal in nature, caused by decreased perfusion of the kidneys due to shock or dehydration.

147–A

Minimal change disease (MCD) is the most common cause of nephrotic syndrome in children, accounting for 80% of cases, followed by focal glomerular sclerosis. Membranous GN is the most common cause in adults, but is much less common in children. Management of uncomplicated nephrotic syndrome includes steroids and salt restriction. Long-term prognosis for MCD is excellent, although the majority (80%) of patients will relapse at least once.

148–D

All of the listed options are possible complications of nephrotic syndrome. Bacterial infections are the most common complication, and spontaneous bacterial peritonitis is the most common infection. Hypercoagulability occurs due to urinary loss of coagulation factors such antithrombin III and protein C. Interestingly, bleeding can also occur due to loss of factors IX, XI, and XII. End-stage renal disease is rare in patients with MCD, but is more common in patients with other causes of nephrotic syndrome.

149–C

Most cases of osteomyelitis in children are hematogenous in origin, and *S. aureus* is the most common pathogen. Immature blood vessels in the metaphysis make children's bones more vulnerable to invasion by bacteria. Most cases occur in children younger than 5 years of age and involve the long bones. The femur and tibia together account for about half of all cases.

150–A

Osteomyelitis is about twice as common in boys as in girls. Trauma or surgery involving the bone predisposes to bacterial invasion by rupturing small blood vessels and creating a favorable environment for bacterial growth. A history of trauma is found in approximately one-third of cases of osteomyelitis. Children with impaired immune function are especially vulnerable to skeletal infection. In particular, children with sickle cell anemia are especially vulnerable because they not only have impaired host defenses from splenic dysfunction, but also suffer bony damage from repeated episodes of vascular compromise.

151–D

All of the listed complications are possible after osteomyelitis. Impaired bone growth occurs if the physis of the bone is damaged by the infection. Close long-term follow up is necessary because these changes may not become apparent for years after the acute infection. Chronic or recurrent skeletal infection occurs in less than 10% of patients. Pathologic fracture may occur due to weakened bone structure, and small children may need to have the limb immobilized to avoid trauma.

152–C

Osteomyelitis in neonates involves more than one bone in almost half of the cases. This is in contrast to older children, in whom involvement of multiple bones is rare. Osteomyelitis is very difficult to diagnose in neonates, because fever is present in less than half of cases, and findings on exam may

ANSWERS

be subtle. The most common bacterial pathogen in neonates, as in older children, is *S. aureus.* Other prominent pathogens include the most common organisms in neonatal sepsis, Group B *Streptococcus* and gram-negative enteric bacilli.

153–B

Febrile seizures can be classified as simple (lasting <10 minutes, maximum 1 episode per 24 hours, and generalized) or complex (>15 minutes, recurring in less than 24 hours, and/or focal). Complex febrile seizures do not predict further complicated febrile seizures, but, in association with family history, may increase the risk for non-febrile seizures or epilepsy.

154–C

Febrile seizures are most likely to occur in children aged 6 months to 5 years, with a peak onset at age 14 to 28 months of age.

155–A

Normal EEGs are expected in patients after a simple febrile seizure and further imaging such as head CT or MRI will not be helpful. The characteristic three-spikes-per-second EEG waveform is associated with petit mal (absence) type seizures. Generalized slowing with or without sharp spikes on EEG may occur as a consequence of global cerebral insult, such as following a hypoxic or ischemic CNS event.

156–C

The developing cortex of the newborn gradually becomes increasingly excitable (and thus more prone to seizures) before "maturing" and becoming less excitable in the second decade of life. Seizures are thus increasingly common during the early years and are then outgrown as the child grows older.

157–C

Coxsackie B virus and echovirus are enteroviruses and are the most common causes of myocarditis in North American children. Coxsackie A virus is responsible for the more common hand-foot-and-mouth disease.

158–A

The hepatic vascular bed is *not* considered a vital end organ. Similarly, the skin, pancreas, and splanchnic vascular beds are also not considered vital end organs.

159–B

The degree of tachycardia is considered the most sensitive measure of intravascular fluid status.

160–A

Glucose infusion is *not* considered a resuscitation medication for septic shock. It is important to treat septic shock with aggressive fluid boluses and the initiation of antibiotics. Soon after hemodynamic stability has been established, appropriate glucose infusions should be administered.

161–E

It is important to understand the various conditions and situations that can mimic physical abuse. Also included are insect bites, impetigo (which can mimic cigarette burns), vasculitic lesions/nevi, and conditions that can mimic or predispose to fracture (e.g., rickets, leukemia, Caffey disease).

162–E

All of the answers are associated with a higher risk for abuse. It should also be noted that abuse is more common in infants and toddlers, but it can occur at *any* age.

163–E

In children younger than 2 years, 80% of head injury deaths result from abuse. Due to the large relative size of the infant head, the pliable skull, lax ligaments, weak cervical spine, and increased plasticity of brain parenchyma, the head is more susceptible to injury from being shaken. Infants may present with profound lethargy, variable tone, posturing, shock, and irritability. Metaphyseal chip fractures result from shearing forces on the corners of long bones.

164–A

Failure to thrive and developmental delay can be the result of all forms of abuse. Accidental burns generally present with a splash and droplet pattern and are usually superficial in nature. Play usually results in bruising on bony protuberances like the elbows and knees. Crying and toilet training are the most common triggers for an abusive incident.

165–C

The primary determinant of neurologic outcome is the length of unconsciousness.

166–D

Because of the uncertainty of possible cervical spine injuries, upon initial evaluation in the field a cervical stabilization collar should *always* be placed. Cranial nerve abnormalities, particularly papillary findings and extraocular movements, can help localize injury and suggest elevated ICP/herniation.

167–C

(A) Subdural bleeds usually appear as crescentic bleeds on CT scan. (B) Subdural bleeds are usually associated with rupture of bridging cortical veins. (C) Epidural bleeds generally occur between the skull and dura. (D) Subdural bleeds generally are associated with intact but altered mental status. (Note: association of impaired mental status followed by a lucid interval and subsequent impairment is not as common in pediatrics as in the adult population.)

168–D

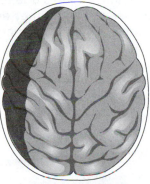

A. Subdural hematoma

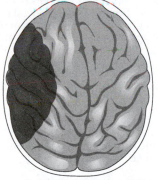

B. Epidural hematoma

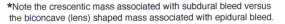

*Note the crescentic mass associated with subdural bleed versus the biconcave (lens) shaped mass associated with epidural bleed.

FIGURE A168 Imaging findings for subdural and epidural bleeds. **(A)** Subdural hematoma. **(B)** Epidural hematoma. Note the crescentic mass associated with subdural bleed versus the biconcave shaped mass associated with epidural bleed. Illustration by Electronic Illustrators Group.

TABLE A168. Differentiating Acute Subdural and Epidural Bleeds

	SUBDURAL	EPIDURAL
Location	Between the dura and arachnoid layers	Between the skull and the dura
Symmetry	Usually bilateral	Usually unilateral
Etiology	Rupture of bridging cortical veins	Rupture of middle meningeal artery or dural veins
Typical injury	Direct trauma or shaking	Direct trauma in the temporal area
Consciousness	Intact but altered	Impaired–lucid–impaired
Common associated findings	Seizures, retinal hemorrhages	Ipsilateral pupillary dilatation, papilledema, contralateral hemiparesis
Appearance on CT with contrast	Crescentic	Biconcave
Prognosis	High morbidity; low mortality	High mortality; low morbidity
Complications	Herniation	Skull fracture; uncal herniation

Used with permission from Marino B, Snead K, McMillan J. Blueprints in Pediatrics, 2nd ed. Malden: Blackwell Science, Inc., 2001: 235.

Cushing's triad (bradycardia, hypertension, and changes in respiration) is associated with *increased* ICP. Posterior auricular bruising (Battle's sign) is associated with basilar skull fractures. Hyperventilation and mannitol help to decrease ICP.

169–C

Intracranial processes include hemorrhage, infarction, infections, and masses. Metabolic derangements, such as hypoglycemia, can be the result of numerous causes. Psychiatric disorders include panic disorders, schizophrenia, and drug withdrawals. Toxic ingestions must always be included in this list. Erythema toxicum neonatorum is a benign rash of the newborn and is not associated with this differential diagnosis.

170–D

Commonly ingested substances have specific antidotes that may aid in the treatment. Diazepam and other benzodiazepines can be treated with flumazenil. Physostigmine is used as an antidote for atropine or antihistamines.

171–B

For acute ingestions, the assessment of ABCs and hemodynamic stability should occur first. Induction of emesis (particularly if the substance was recently ingested), usually with ipecac syrup, can be quite helpful. This mode of therapy is losing favor, but can be helpful in immediate home therapy with a known ingested substance. Activated charcoal can help to bind to the offending substance and expedite its proper elimination. Gastric lavage, used less frequently in cases of acute ingestion, may help to remove and dilute stomach contents. Although ABCs should always be assessed first, the next sequence of treatments is generally determined by the nature of the poisoning. Although seizures may initially be present a patient with an acute ingestion, EEG plays no role in the initial management of an acute poisoning. Poison Control hotlines are an invaluable resource and should be rapidly accessed by caregivers and healthcare providers in these situations.

172–C

Hydrocarbons in the lung trigger a profound inflammatory reaction and can result in a chemical pneumonitis. Preventing aspiration is the primary goal in hydrocarbon ingestion. Activated charcoal is a useful method of treatment; however, its use is limited in the ingestion of certain substances (such as alcohol, hydrocarbons, iron, and lithium). Mydriasis, tachycardia, and hypertension are usually characteristics of sympathomimetic substances. Cholinergic substances generally are associated with other symptoms, such as meiosis, salivation, and lacrimation. Home safety and education are the most important tools in preventing ingestions.

173–C

Drastic weight loss is not typical of patients with bulimia nervosa, who tend to be of normal weight or slightly obese. The other symptoms listed are all characteristic of bulimia nervosa.

174–D

All of the disorders listed are possible consequences of AN. Cardiac arrhythmias, which may be fatal, include supraventricular dysrhythmias, T wave inversion, and prolonged QT. Due to the high likelihood of osteoporosis in patients with AN, many practitioners recommend bone density studies in these patients to document the degree of bone loss. Osteoporosis is usually reversible with nutrition. Chronic inability to maintain normal weight occurs in 15% to 20% of patients.

175–D

Although sports-related injuries are common in malnourished female athletes due to nutritional deficiencies and overtraining, they are not part of the female athlete triad. The triad includes anorexia, amenorrhea, and osteoporosis. Amenorrhea is thought to be due to a combination of weight loss and hypothalamic-pituitary disturbances, and persists in 25% of patients after restoration of healthy weight.

TABLE A172. Signs, Symptoms, and Treatment of Specific Pediatric Poisonings

SUBSTANCE	CLINICAL MANIFESTATIONS	ANTIDOTE/TREATMENT
Acetaminophen	Nausea/vomiting, anorexia, pallor, diaphoresis; may progress over days to jaundice, abdominal pain, liver failure	A: N-acetylcysteine T: gastric emptying if <2 hours since ingestion; activated charcoal if <4 hours since ingestion. Draw blood level at 4 hours and use available nomogram to assess risk of hepatotoxicity. If toxic, start oral N-acetylcysteine and continue for 72 hours.
Anticholinergics (atropine, tricyclic antidepressants, antihistamines, phenothiazides)	Fever, mydriasis, flushing, dry skin, tachycardia, hypertension, cardiac arrhythmias, delirium, psychosis, convulsion, coma	A: physostigmine for atropine and antihistamines A: $NaCO_2$, $MgSO_4$ for tricyclic antidepressants
Cholinergics (organophosphates and other pesticides)	Nausea/vomiting, sweating, meiosis, salivation, lacrimation, bronchorrhea, urination, defecation, weakness, muscle fasciculation, paralysis, confusion, coma	A: pralidoxime chloride T: gastric lavage, activated charcoal; prophylactic atropine
Opiates	Pinpoint pupils, bradypnea, hypotension, hypothermia, stupor, coma	A: naloxone T: evaluate and secure airway as needed; gastrointestinal decontamination if appropriate; naloxone
Sedatives/hypnotics	Nystagmus, meiosis or mydriasis, hypothermia, hypotension, bradypnea, confusion, ataxia, coma	A: flumazenil for benzodiazepines T: evaluate and secure airway if needed; maintain hemodynamic stability; activated charcoal with cathartic; supportive care

Modified from Marino B, Snead K, McMillan J. Blueprints in Pediatrics, 2nd ed. Malden: Blackwell Science, Inc., 2001: 7.

176–B

Although previously reported primarily in middle and upper socioeconomic groups, AN is now recognized to occur in all socioeconomic and racial/ethnic groups. Approximately 10% of those affected are males. Bulimia nervosa is approximately five times as common as anorexia nervosa, which occurs in about 1% of females 14 to 18 years of age. The incidence of eating disorders has been steadily increasing in the last 20 years, and is greater among high risk groups such as college students, gymnasts and other athletes, and those with a history of sexual abuse.

177–D

Treatment of leukemia, which is initiated in the hospital, includes treating the complications from the disease at presentation (transfusing blood products, stabilizing electrolytes, restoring nutrition, treating infection), treating the leukemia itself (specific regimens vary by institution, but include chemotherapeutic phases of induction, consolidation, and maintenance therapy), and managing the complications of therapy. The overall cure rate for childhood ALL is 80%. Bone marrow transplant is indicated only for patients who do not respond to standard treatment.

178–D

All of the listed conditions are common in children receiving chemotherapy for ALL. Children being treated for ALL are carefully monitored for electrolyte and metabolic disturbances, which can occur due to the release of potassium, phosphate, and purines from the large burden of malignant cells being killed by chemotherapy. Bone marrow suppression results in depression of all cell lines, and children often need replacement of red cells and platelets to prevent severe anemia and bleeding. Neutropenia resulting from chemotherapy places these children at high risk for invasive infection and sepsis, and they must be monitored carefully for fever and any other signs of infection while they are immunosuppressed. Alopecia is nearly universal during induction, but resolves in the later phases of treatment.

179–C

Brain tumors in children, in contrast to those in adults, are usually infratentorial. CNS tumors are the most common solid tumors of childhood.

Symptoms are often a clue to the location of the tumor. For example, ataxia and nystagmus suggest a cerebellar mass, whereas hyperreflexia and multiple cranial nerve deficits suggest a brainstem lesion. Pituitary, hypothalamic, or pineal tumors may present with growth or endocrine disturbances. It is important to keep in mind, however, that the early symptoms of brain tumors, such as headache, personality changes, or vomiting, are often nonspecific, and may initially be dismissed as a viral illness. Making the diagnosis requires maintaining a high degree of suspicion when a child's symptoms are unusual, prolonged, or are unresponsive to treatment.

180–B

Most (~60%) childhood lymphomas are non-Hodgkin lymphomas (NHL). Lymphoma is the third most common childhood malignancy, accounting for 10% to 15% of pediatric cancers. At presentation, the peripheral blood counts are usually normal unless the bone marrow is involved. NHL with >25% blasts is classified as ALL. The overall survival is ~70%, with the most favorable outcome for early stage NHL.

181–B

In most cases of FTT, the cause is primarily nonorganic. About one-fourth of cases involve a combination of organic and nonorganic factors. Most children with FTT have a good prognosis with respect to weight gain and growth. However, approximately one-fourth of these patients remain small. Cognitive function may be impaired and behavioral problems are more common in patients with severe or long-standing FTT.

182–A

Poverty, not middle or high socioeconomic status, is a risk factor for failure to thrive (FTT). Prenatal factors such as prematurity and intrauterine growth retardation are also associated with a higher risk of FTT. Children with chronic disease, especially cardiac or neurologic disease, are at risk for both organic and nonorganic forms of poor growth. Social stressors such as domestic violence, financial difficulties, and mental illness all contribute to a child's risk of FTT.

183–B

In the infant or child with nonorganic failure to thrive, as in the case above, head circumference

ANSWERS

and length should be preserved. Symmetric decrease in all of the growth parameters should suggest an organic cause. Successful weight gain with refeeding, normal laboratory tests and normal physical examination all support a nonorganic cause of FTT.

184–C

The nutritional needs of a healthy 4-month-old child are met adequately by sufficient quantities of breast milk or formula alone. Additional fluids, such as water or supplements, are unnecessary. Around 4 to 6 months, rice cereal is often introduced, followed by cooked, pureed baby foods. Fresh fruits and vegetables and cow's milk are not recommended until 1 year of age. During the first year of life, a growing infant requires 100 to 120 calories/kg per day for proper growth. Breast milk and formula contain about 20 calories per oz.

185–C

The throat culture is the gold standard for diagnosis. Although diagnosis of an acute GAS pharyngitis is often made clinically, based on history, physical findings, and experience, studies show that it is more accurate and cost-effective to use laboratory tests such as the rapid antigen test ("rapid Strep") combined with throat culture to guide therapy. Both of these tests rely on the quality of the sample for adequate sensitivity. The rapid antigen test is specific, but its sensitivity varies from institution to institution. Therefore, a throat culture should always be sent along with the rapid antigen test to ensure adequate sensitivity. Because protection against ARF is achieved if treatment is begun within 10 days of the start of the infection, results of the throat culture can be obtained before the onset of treatment. However, many physicians prefer to start therapy based on clinical suspicion and rapid Strep results, and stop treatment if the culture is negative. Treatment does *not* shorten severity or duration of symptoms, but does help to prevent both suppurative and nonsuppurative consequences.

186–D

Positive culture for GAS is not considered a major criterion for the diagnosis of ARF, although it is supportive of the diagnosis. The major and minor criteria for diagnosis of ARF, known as the Jones criteria, are listed in the table below. ARF is an immune-mediated condition that occurs 3 to 4 weeks after an acute GAS infection, and involves the tissues of the heart, joints, and brain. Its prevention is an important reason to treat acute GAS pharyngitis. Although rheumatic fever has declined greatly in prevalence since the initiation of widespread use of penicillin to treat GAS infections, it still exists; thus, it should be kept in mind as part of the differential diagnosis in a case such as this one. Treatment of ARF includes antibiotics, anti-inflammatory drugs and cardiac management. Patients with ARF should also be treated with prophylactic penicillin to prevent subsequent GAS infections, which are associated with recurrence.

TABLE A186. Revised Jones Criteria for the Diagnosis of Acute Rheumatic Fever

Major manifestations
Carditis
Polyarthritis
Chorea
Erythema marginatum
Subcutaneous nodules

Minor manifestations
Clinical
Fever
Arthralgia
Previous rheumatic fever/rheumatic heart disease
Laboratory
Acute-phase reaction[a]
Prolonged PR interval

Additional criteria
Supporting evidence of preceding streptococcal infection (increased ASO or other streptococcal antibodies), *OR*
Positive throat culture for group A streptococci, *OR*
Recent scarlet fever

[a]Elevated serum erythrocyte sedimentation rate (ESR), C-reactive protein; leukocytosis.

Used with permission from Marino B, Snead K, McMillan J. Blueprints in Pediatrics, 2nd ed. Malden: Blackwell Science, Inc., 2001: 155.

187–B

PSGN is most commonly associated with GAS skin infections. Unlike ARF, it is *not* preventable by antibiotic treatment. PSGN is a postinfectious, immune-mediated condition in which immune complexes deposit in the kidneys causing acute glomerulonephritis. The development of hematuria, hypertension, or nephrotic syndrome (edema, proteinuria, oliguria) in a child who has a recent history of skin infection or sore throat should raise suspicion of PSGN. Management is supportive, and includes penicillin and antihypertensives if needed. Most cases resolve without permanent morbidity.

188–C

Toxic shock syndrome, which results from a toxin mediated by strains of *S. aureus* (although a similar syndrome can result from streptococcal toxins as well), is a medical emergency. The rash is a diffuse erythema, like a sunburn, and is accompanied by hypotension, high fever, conjunctival and oral erythema, and multiple organ system involvement. Although historically associated with tampon use, the syndrome can also occur as a result of infection in the bone or skin. Treatment consists of antibiotics and supportive care.

189–A

Platelet transfusion may be indicated to help stop acute bleeding in severe cases of ITP, but is not indicated in this case. The management of ITP is directed toward avoiding the rare but serious complications of internal or cerebral hemorrhage by slowing the destruction of platelets and avoiding trauma. Medical treatment, which is indicated if clinically significant bleeding is present or if platelet counts are below 20,000, may include high-dose steroids or IVIG. These measures temporarily raise platelet counts due to decreased clearance of antibody-coated platelets, but they do not shorten the duration of antibody production or the long-term outcome of ITP. Due to this patient's low platelet count, most physicians would treat him with steroids or IVIG until his platelet count climbs above 30,000. He can then be managed as an outpatient with regular checks of platelet count to document recovery. He should avoid contact sports and activities that may result in trauma, such as bike riding or rollerblading, until his platelet count is at least 70,000. Most cases of ITP (~80%) resolve spontaneously in 6 months and never recur; the remainder may become relapsing or chronic. Rarely, ITP may be the presenting symptom of HIV infection or an autoimmune disease such as systemic lupus erythematosus (SLE).

190–C

A toxic-appearing child with a petechial rash is septic until proven otherwise, so the choice of antibiotics should cover a broad range of gram-positive and gram-negative organisms, as well as have adequate penetration into the CNS. Ceftriaxone is a good choice for this purpose. Vancomycin should be added in any sick child who may have infection with *S. pneumoniae*, to cover the small but significant percentage of these organisms that are drug resistant. The most feared cause of this clinical picture is meningococcemia. Children with this infection deteriorate rapidly, and may die despite rapid intervention with appropriate support and antibiotic therapy. Other bacterial causes of sepsis and petechiae in children out of the neonatal period include *S. pneumoniae*, *H. influenzae* type B, and gram-negative organisms such as *E. coli*.

191–C

Chronic ITP is more common in older children (>10 years), and is defined as thrombocytopenia persisting for longer than 6 months. It is treated with repeated doses of IVIG, or with splenectomy, which induces remission in 70% to 80% of cases. In refractory cases with uncontrolled bleeding, immunosuppressive drugs, plasmapheresis, or drugs that inhibit fibrinolysis have been used.

192–B

Heart murmurs are *not* associated with HSP, a systemic vasculitis most common in children 3 to 7 years of age. HSP is a clinically diagnosed syndrome consisting of a characteristic rash, as well as a variety of associated features. The rash may be urticarial, papular, or petechial at onset, then coalesces into larger purpuric areas. It is typically located on the buttocks and legs, but may involve the trunk, arms, or face. Other commonly associated features include fever, abdominal pain, joint pain, scrotal swelling, and hematuria. Rarely, renal failure, seizures, or intussusception may occur as a result of HSP. Treatment is mainly supportive, with adequate hydration and careful monitoring for signs of significant renal, GI, or CNS manifestations. Use of steroids in controversial, but may be indicated in treatment of GI or CNS symptoms, and in severe renal disease.

ANSWERS

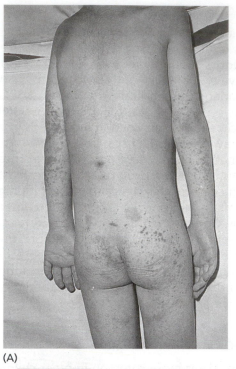

(A)

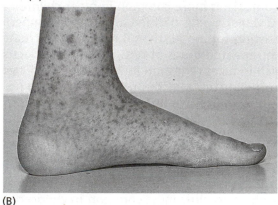

(B)

FIGURE A192 Typical palpable, nonblanching rash of Henoch-Schönlein purpura (HSP). Used with permission from Rudolf M, Levene M. Paediatrics and Child Health. Oxford: Blackwell Science, Ltd., 1999: 200.

193–D

Meningitis does not generally cause a facial cellulitis. However, cellulitis may occur from the spread of bacteria from other underlying infections, such as dental infection or sinusitis, mastoiditis, osteomyelitis, or septic arthritis. A CT scan or MRI can help to document involvement of the underlying structures in unclear cases. Cellulitis arising from sinus, bone, or dental infection is managed by treating the underlying infection. Bacteria in the blood can also penetrate the face and orbital area, causing facial or orbital cellulitis. This type of hematogenously spread cellulitis, frequently caused by *S. pneumoniae* or

H. influenzae, is much more common in children prior to the advent of widespread vaccination for *H. influenzae*. New vaccines against *S. pneumoniae* may further rarify this dangerous entity.

194–A

Impetigo is a superficial infection of the skin. It is most commonly caused by staphylococcal species, but streptococcal species may also be present. Impetigo occurs in two forms: bullous and nonbullous. Bullous impetigo, most common in newborns, is always caused by *S. aureus*, and produces thin-walled bullae over an erythematous base that produce a clear, thin coating when they rupture. Nonbullous impetigo is a common and relatively benign infection of the skin that may be caused by staphylococcal *or* streptococcal species, and typically involves painless, small (5-mm) vesicles and pustules that rupture, producing a golden crusted coating over an ulcerated base. Limited nonbullous impetigo can be treated with topical mupirocin ointment, whereas bullous or extensive nonbullous impetigo is treated with an oral antibiotic effective against *Staphylococcus* and *Streptococcus*, such as a first-generation cephalosporin.

195–A

Fever is generally not a clinical feature of anaphylaxis, which is a rapid and life-threatening systemic allergic reaction. Impending airway compromise may be heralded by lip or tongue swelling, wheeze, dry cough, or difficulty speaking. Hypotension is an early sign of the circulatory effects of anaphylaxis, which may progress to shock if not identified and treated early. Urticaria, abdominal pain, and diarrhea are other signs of anaphylaxis. Any suspicion of airway inflammation in a patient with an allergic reaction should be treated immediately with subcutaneous epinephrine, and the patient should be taken to an area where the airway can be secured if necessary. Intravenous steroids and antihistamines may also be of benefit. Circulatory complications should be managed as necessary with fluid resuscitation and cardiovascular support.

196–D

Conjunctivitis should *not* be accompanied by severe pain or swelling, changes in vision, poor pupillary reactivity, or fever. The presence of any of these findings should prompt consideration of iritis, corneal abrasion, or a more severe eye infection. Conjunctivitis is a common condition in children that may be infectious, allergic, or chemical in origin. It is characterized by diffuse injection of the sclera and conjunctivae, mild lid swelling, watery or purulent discharge, and eye itching or discomfort. Although most infective conjunctivitis, whether of bacterial or viral origins, will resolve on its own in 4 to 5 days, day-care centers and schools often require that the child receive treatment before returning to school. Topical erythromycin, tobramycin, or sulfacetamide drops are usually sufficient treatment. Allergic conjunctivitis can be treated with mild vasoconstricting eye drops if the discomfort is severe.

197–D

The cause of eczema is unknown, but both hereditary and environmental factors seem to play a role. Seventy percent of children with eczema have a family history of atopy (food allergies, hayfever or asthma), and 50% to 80% go on to develop allergic rhinitis or asthma themselves. Eczema has been described as "an itch that rashes," which suggests that the skin manifestations are primarily a result of scratching the affected area, rather than the underlying pathologic process. The rash tends to have a waxing and waning course, typified by flares of symptoms that may be triggered by irritants such as certain foods, chemicals in soaps, lotions or detergents, pets, smoking, or dry weather.

198–A

Bathing in hot water and scrubbing with soap will actually exacerbate dryness and itchiness of the skin. Tepid water baths are recommended, and additives such as oatmeal may be helpful for additional relief. An oral antihistamine such as diphenhydramine can help reduce itching, but may cause drowsiness during the day. Trimming fingernails short prevents excoriation of the skin, and the use of cotton gloves at night may further reduce damage from scratching. Regular moisturization, especially immediately after bathing, hydrates and heals the skin.

199–C

Ringworm, or *tinea corporis*, produces an annular lesion with central clearing. Topical clotrimazole or miconazole, applied for 4 to 6 weeks, is usually effective in treating this condition. *Tinea capitis*, which is characterized by round scaly patches of alopecia on the scalp or base of the neck, should be treated with oral griseofulvin or another oral antifungal agent, as topical agents are usually ineffective. *Scabies*, a highly contagious mite infection, is characterized by pruritic linear streaks of papules and pustules with surrounding erythema. Treatment consists of application of 5% permethrin cream to the entire body of the patient and close contacts, and washing of all sheets and clothing to prevent reinfection. *Seborrheic dermatitis*, also known as cradle cap, affects two pediatric age groups: infants and adolescents. In infants it consists of a greasy yellow scale that starts at the scalp and may spread to involve the face and intertriginous areas. Treatment consists of a tar-based shampoo or mild topical steroid. *Psoriasis* typically appears as sharply demarginated plaques with silvery scale occurring on knees and elbows.

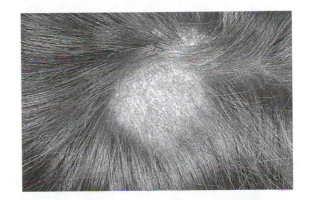

FIGURE A199-1 Tinea capitis. A circumscribed patch of hair loss is seen with patchy scaling of the scalp. Used with permission from Rudolf M, Levene M. Paediatrics and Child Health. Oxford: Blackwell Science, Ltd., 1999: 210.

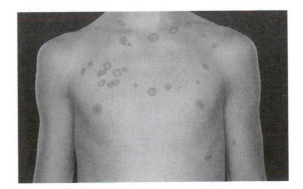

FIGURE A199-2 Tinea corporis. Typical ring-like patches with central clearing on the trunk. Used with permission from Rudolf M, Levene M. Paediatrics and Child Health. Oxford: Blackwell Science, Ltd., 1999: 210.

ANSWERS

200–B

Growth retardation is generally not considered a side effect of topical steroid therapy. Children who require frequent or chronic courses of oral steroids for very severe eczema, asthma, or other conditions, however, may experience some growth delay. Topical steroids may cause thinning of the skin with prolonged use, and should not be applied to the eyelids and other areas of delicate skin. Low to high potencies of topical steroids are available, and should be selected based on the location and severity of the rash. In general the lowest potency agent that controls the patient's symptoms should be employed, and prolonged use should be avoided.

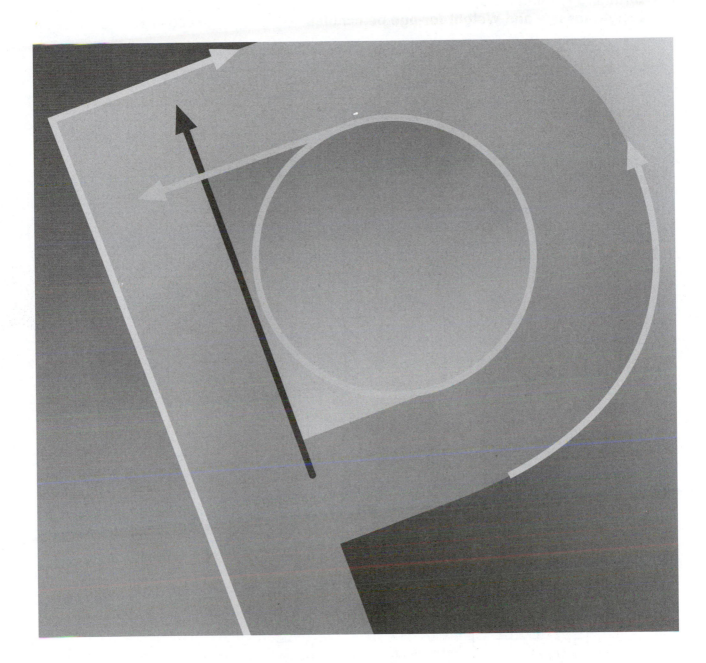

APPENDIX I:
GROWTH CHARTS

Birth to 36 months: Boys
Length-for-age and Weight-for-age percentiles

NAME _____

RECORD # _____

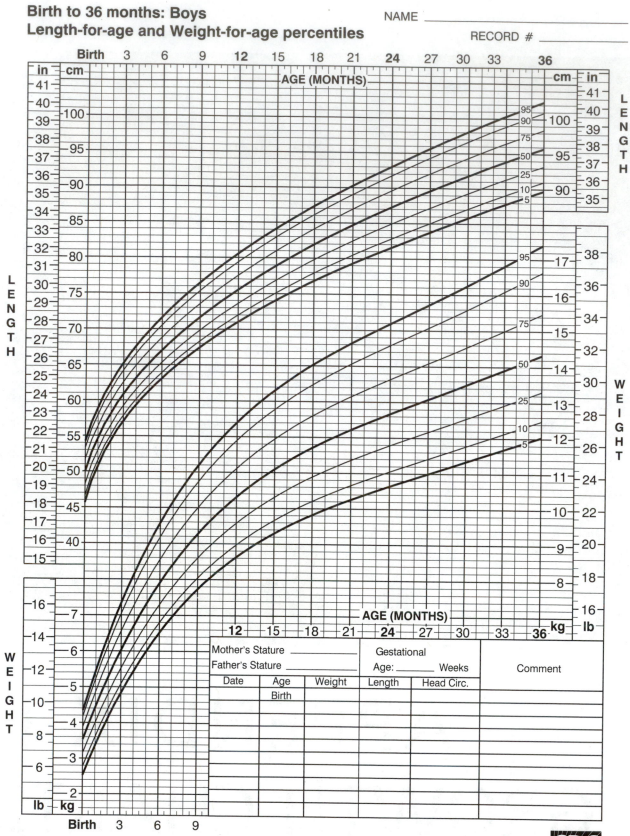

Revised April 20, 2001.
SOURCE: Developed by the National Center for Health Statistics in collaboration with
the National Center for Chronic Disease Prevention and Health Promotion (2000).
http://www.cdc.gov/growthcharts

Birth to 36 months: Boys
Head circumference-for-age and
Weight-for-length percentiles

NAME _____

RECORD # _____

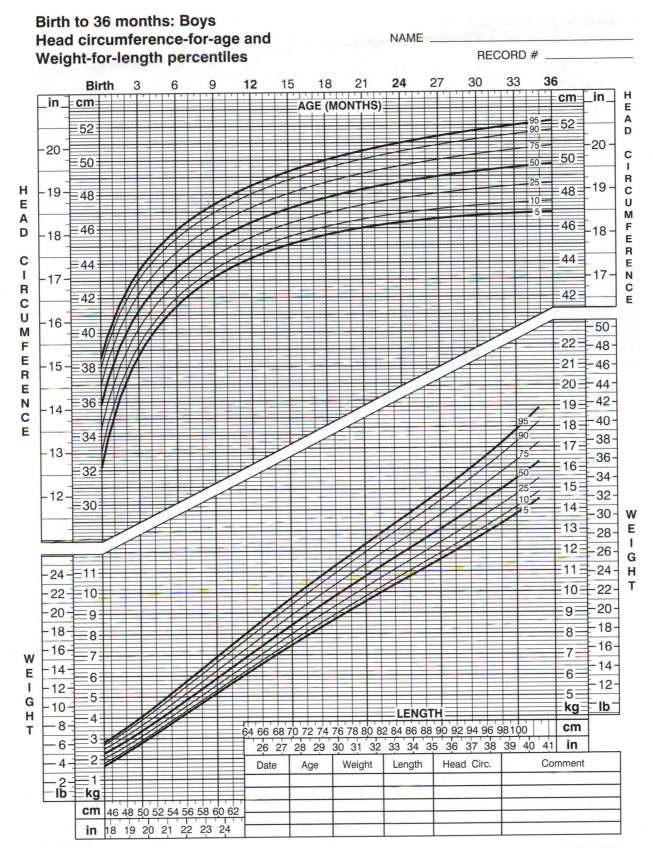

SOURCE: Developed by the National Center for Health Statistics in collaboration with
the National Center for Chronic Disease Prevention and Health Promotion (2000).
http://www.cdc.gov/growthcharts

Birth to 36 months: Girls
Length-for-age and Weight-for-age percentiles

NAME _____

RECORD # _____

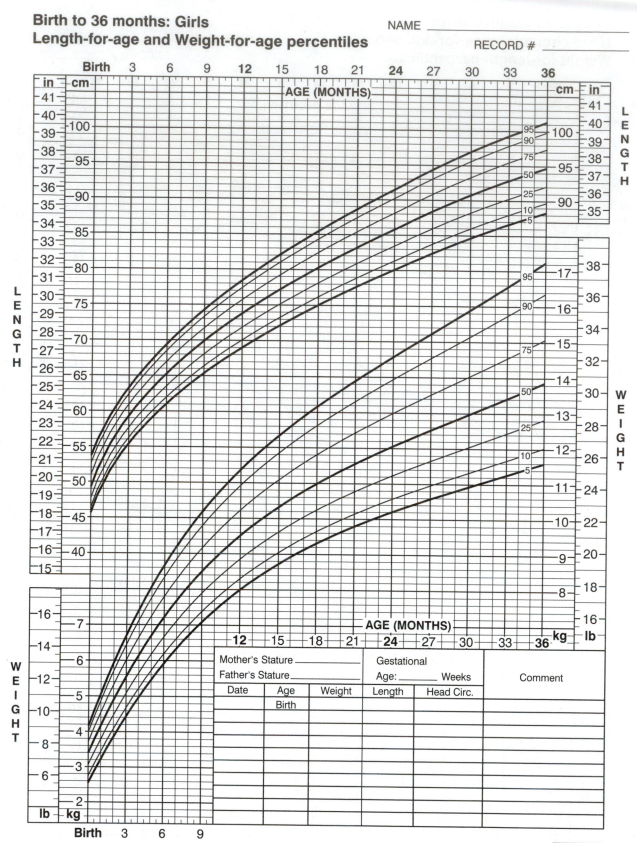

Revised April 20, 2001.
SOURCE: Developed by the National Center for Health Statistics in collaboration with
the National Center for Chronic Disease Prevention and Health Promotion (2000).
http://www.cdc.gov/growthcharts

Birth to 36 months: Girls
Head circumference-for-age and
Weight-for-length percentiles

NAME _____

RECORD # _____

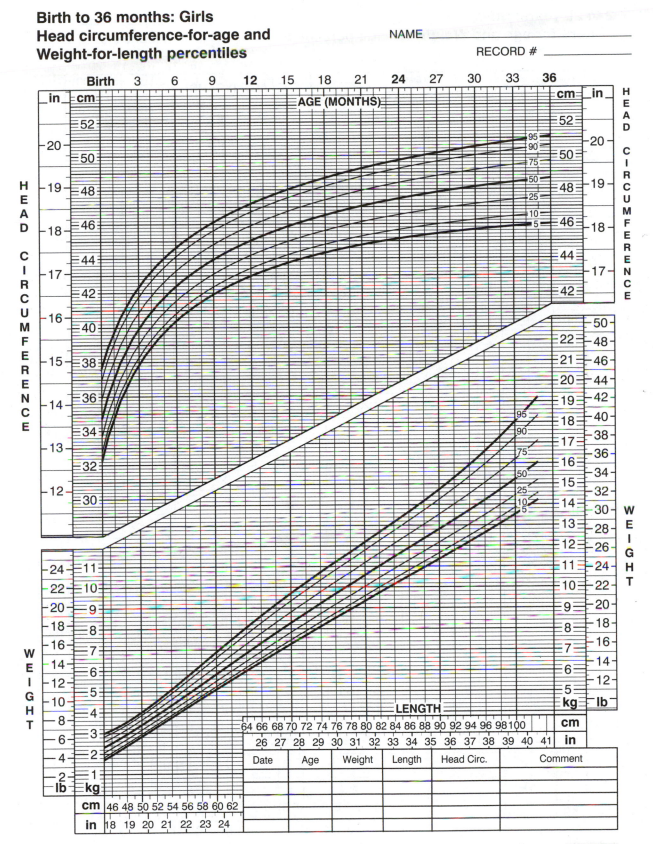

SOURCE: Developed by the National Center for Health Statistics in collaboration with
the National Center for Chronic Disease Prevention and Health Promotion (2000).
http://www.cdc.gov/growthcharts

2 to 20 years: Boys
Stature-for-age and Weight-for-age percentiles

NAME _____

RECORD # _____

Mother's Stature _____ Father's Stature _____

Date	Age	Weight	Stature	BMI*

*To Calculate BMI: Weight (kg) ÷ Stature (cm) ÷ Stature (cm) x 10,000
or Weight (lb) ÷ Stature (in) ÷ Stature (in) x 703

AGE (YEARS)

STATURE

WEIGHT

Revised and corrected November 28, 2000.

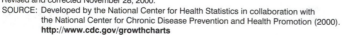

SOURCE: Developed by the National Center for Health Statistics in collaboration with
the National Center for Chronic Disease Prevention and Health Promotion (2000).
http://www.cdc.gov/growthcharts

2 to 20 years: Boys
Body mass index-for-age percentiles

NAME _____

RECORD # _____

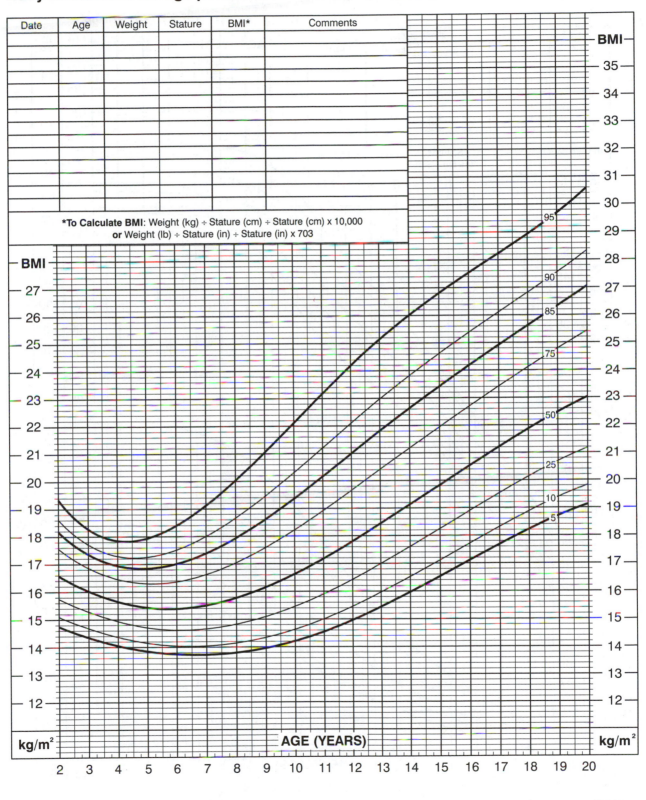

Date	Age	Weight	Stature	BMI*	Comments

*To Calculate BMI: Weight (kg) ÷ Stature (cm) ÷ Stature (cm) x 10,000
or Weight (lb) ÷ Stature (in) ÷ Stature (in) x 703

BMI

AGE (YEARS)

kg/m²   kg/m²

SOURCE: Developed by the National Center for Health Statistics in collaboration with
the National Center for Chronic Disease Prevention and Health Promotion (2000).
http://www.cdc.gov/growthcharts

141

2 to 20 years: Girls
Stature-for-age and Weight-for-age percentiles

NAME _____

RECORD # _____

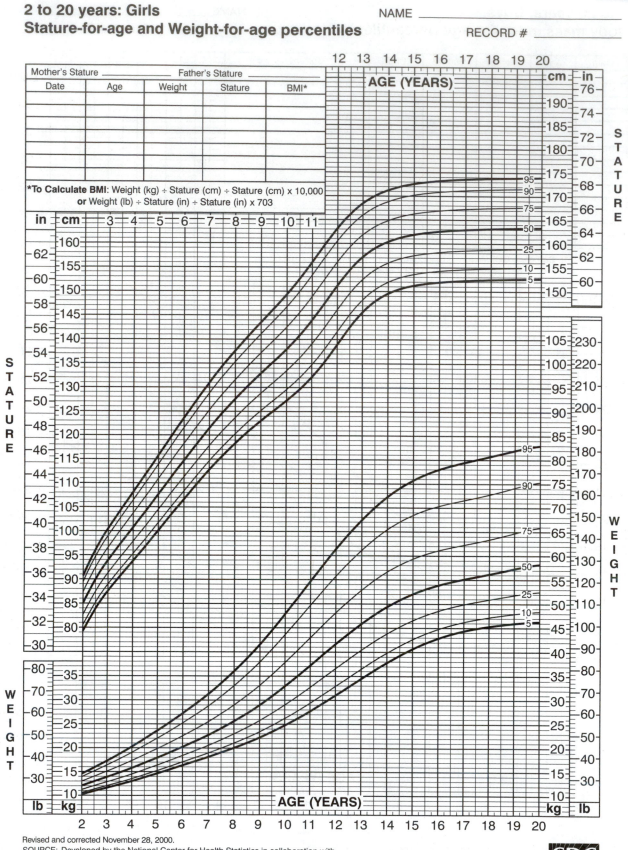

Revised and corrected November 28, 2000.

SOURCE: Developed by the National Center for Health Statistics in collaboration with
the National Center for Chronic Disease Prevention and Health Promotion (2000).
http://www.cdc.gov/growthcharts

CDC

2 to 20 years: Girls
Body mass index-for-age percentiles

NAME _____

RECORD # _____

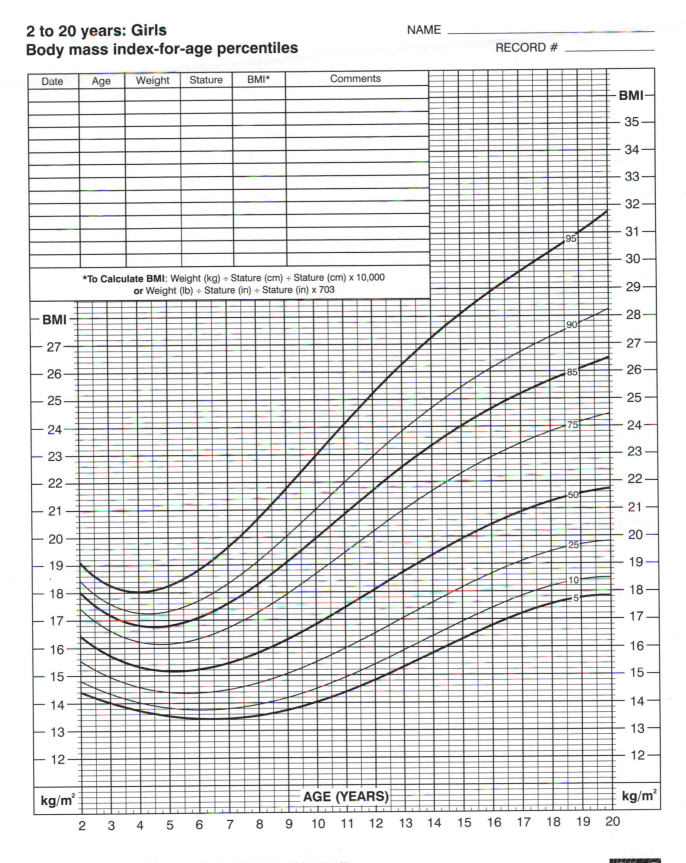

Date	Age	Weight	Stature	BMI*	Comments

*To Calculate BMI: Weight (kg) ÷ Stature (cm) ÷ Stature (cm) x 10,000
or Weight (lb) ÷ Stature (in) ÷ Stature (in) x 703

AGE (YEARS)

SOURCE: Developed by the National Center for Health Statistics in collaboration with
the National Center for Chronic Disease Prevention and Health Promotion (2000).
http://www.cdc.gov/growthcharts

INDEX

INDEX

INDEX

"coffee grounds," 58
confusion with, 84
diarrhea with, 52–53, 119
fever with, 4–5, 105–106
intussusception with, 119
irritability with, 56–57, 119–120
nonbilious, 54
pneumonia with, 18

for poisoning, 127–128
pyloric stenosis with, 54–55, 55f, 119

Walk, refusal to, 68–77
Weight loss, 88–93
  pallor with, 90–91
Wheezing, 16–17, 110–111, 111f
  croup with, 109–110

rash with, 22–23, 112
Wilson's disease, 113
Wolff-Parkinson-White (WPW) syndrome, 115

Yersinia enterocolitica, 48

Zoster, 11, 98, 108f